Human Dignity and Assisted Death

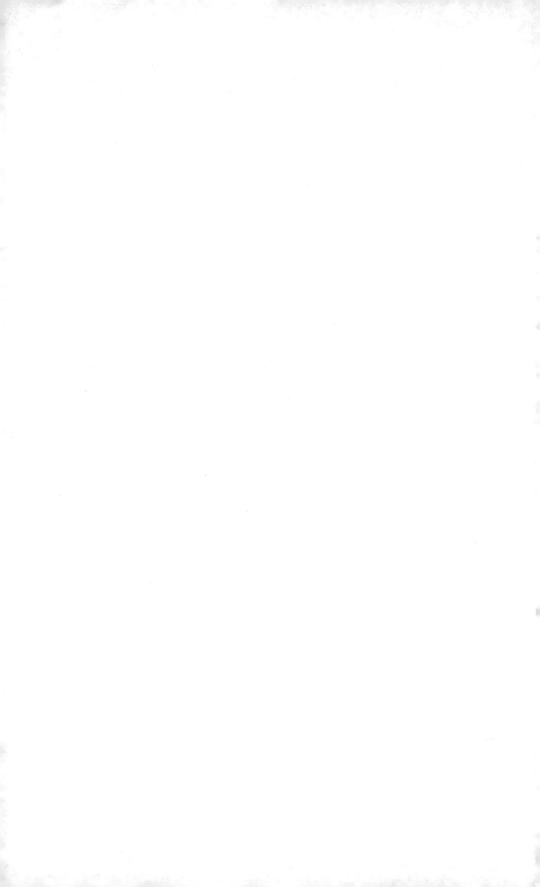

Human Dignity and
Assisted Death

Edited by SEBASTIAN MUDERS

Oxford University Press is a department of the University of Oxford. It furthers
the University's objective of excellence in research, scholarship, and education
by publishing worldwide. Oxford is a registered trade mark of Oxford University
Press in the UK and certain other countries.

Published in the United States of America by Oxford University Press
198 Madison Avenue, New York, NY 10016, United States of America.

Library of Congress Cataloging-in-Publication Data
Names: Muders, Sebastian, editor.
Title: Human dignity and assisted death / edited by Sebastian Muders.
Description: New York, NY : Oxford University Press, 2018. |
Includes bibliographical references and index.
Identifiers: LCCN 2017012754 | ISBN 9780190675967 (hardcover : alk. paper) |
ISBN 9780190675974 (updf)
Subjects: | MESH: Right to Die—ethics | Suicide, Assisted—ethics | Personhood |
Euthanasia—ethics | Attitude to Death
Classification: LCC R726 | NLM W 85.5 | DDC 179.7—dc23
LC record available at https://lccn.loc.gov/2017012754

9 8 7 6 5 4 3 2 1
Printed by Sheridan Books, Inc., United States of America

CONTENTS

ACKNOWLEDGMENTS

My first and special thanks goes to two colleagues without whom this volume would not have been possible. Many of the chapters in this book were first presented during an international workshop titled "The Role of Human Dignity in Assisted Suicide," which took place in Zurich in early February 2014. In the course of the workshop, two of the participants, Margaret Battin and Jeff McMahan, suggested that it might be a worthwhile enterprise to bring together the different papers and arguments into a collected volume, complemented by further invited contributions. Both have supported this project with their expertise, energy, and advice during all the stages of preparation, and I am deeply grateful for their wholehearted support. I further thank the Swiss National Science Foundation for its financial support of my research, and I thank my colleagues and friends at the Centre for Ethics in Zurich for providing such a stimulating and friendly atmosphere. Finally, my thanks to all the contributors of the volume for their splendid texts and to Andrew Ward and Isla Ng at Oxford University Press for their patience and assistance.

CONTRIBUTORS

Margaret P. Battin is Distinguished Professor of Philosophy and Adjunct Professor of Internal Medicine, Division of Medical Ethics, University of Utah, Provo, Utah.

Holger Baumann is Post-Doctoral Fellow at the Ethics Research Institute, Philosophy Department, University of Zurich, Zurich, Switzerland.

Michael Cholbi is Professor of Philosophy at California State Polytechnic University, Pomona, California.

Rebecca Dresser is Daniel Noyes Kirby Professor of Law Emerita, Washington University in St. Louis, St. Louis, Missouri.

William J. FitzPatrick is the Gideon Webster Burbank Professor of Intellectual and Moral Philosophy at the University of Rochester, Rochester, New York.

Robert P. George is the McCormick Professor of Jurisprudence at Princeton University and the founding director of the James Madison Program in American Ideals and Institutions, Princeton, New Jersey.

Luke Gormally is Director Emeritus of the Linacre Centre for Healthcare Ethics, London, UK.

Christopher Kaczor is Professor of Philosophy at Loyola Marymount University, Los Angeles, California.

Jeff McMahan is White's Professor of Moral Philosophy at Oxford University and a fellow of Corpus Christi College, Oxford, UK.

Sebastian Muders is Post-Doctoral Fellow at the Ethics Research Institute, Philosophy Department, University of Zurich, Zurich, Switzerland.

Peter Schaber is Professor of Applied Ethics at the Ethics Research Institute, University of Zurich, Zurich, Switzerland.

Ralf Stoecker is Professor of Practical Philosophy in the Department of Philosophy, University of Bielefeld, Bielefeld, Germany.

L. W. Sumner is University Professor Emeritus in the Department of Philosophy at the University of Toronto, Toronto, Ontario, Canada.

David Wasserman is a faculty member in the Department of Bioethics, National Institutes of Health, Bethesda, Maryland.

CHAPTER 1 | Introduction

SEBASTIAN MUDERS

The Role of Human Dignity in Assisted Death

For more than thirty years, assisted suicide and euthanasia, which are often combined in the term "assisted death" or "assisted dying," have been heavily debated in practical ethics. The topic is a particularly pressing issue of our time because an increase in wealth and medical progress has led to a rapidly aging population—in the Western Hemisphere as well as in Asia and other areas of the world. Moral philosophy has yet to provide a satisfactory discussion of the central dimensions of this urgent problem.

Despite the wide-ranging, complicated philosophical debate on this question, which has given rise to seemingly irreconcilably opposing sides, human dignity is hardly ever mentioned in the discussion. Even in book-length monographs dedicated to this topic, one often hardly finds more than a passing reference to dignity.[1] Whether in arguments for the right to a self-determined end or for the intrinsic worth of human life, dignity tends to be mentioned only briefly and without sufficient analysis of its meaning or moral significance.

This is surprising, for specifically in the public debate on the advantages and disadvantages of assisted death, human dignity, far from being absent, is quite frequently referred to. As several studies have shown, terminally

---

[1] Examples include Margaret Battin, *Ending Life* (New York: Oxford University Press, 2005); Neil Gorsuch, *The Future of Assisted Suicide and Euthanasia* (Princeton, NJ: Princeton University Press, 2006); Jeff McMahan, *The Ethics of Killing: Problems at the Margins of Life* (New York: Oxford University Press, 2002); Graig Paterson, *Physician-Assisted Suicide and Euthanasia: A Natural Law Ethics Approach* (Aldershot, UK: Ashgate, 2008); and Leonard W. Sumner, *Assisted Death: A Study in Ethics and Law* (New York: Oxford University Press, 2011).

ill patients, their physicians, and their relatives alike regularly mention concerns about the patient's dignity when they are asked what they are most worried about concerning his or her condition.[2] Whatever one might think about dignity in general, it is clearly influential in medical contexts. This phenomenon needs to be explained: What is dignity's exact role in these contexts, and to what extent can it be justified?

Since the academic use of the notion of dignity is hardly ever explained in the context of assisted death, it arouses much suspicion, both in this debate and in bioethics more generally. Ruth Macklin's famous claim that dignity is a "useless concept" and Steven Pinker's verdict about the "stupidity of dignity" mark the more influential voices in a choir of skeptics.[3]

Then again, this choir also has provoked much resistance in recent years:[4] Nowadays, almost everybody is inclined to think that dignity, at least generally, can be made more precise in order to be usefully employed in bioethical debates. Likewise, as the ongoing debate has revealed, there seem to be no easy synonyms at hand to encompass the full spectrum of goods that human dignity is tailor-made to articulate, such as human life, autonomy, and self-respect.

Needless to say, this does not mean that a settled theory or conception of human dignity is available, or that there is an unchallenged set of opinions about how this conception can inform certain arguments and

---

[2] See Harvey Max Chochinov et al., "Dignity in the Terminally Ill: A Cross-Sectional, Cohort Study," *The Lancet* 360, no. 9350 (2002): 2026–2030; Sabrina Cipolletta and Nadia Oprandi, "What Is a Good Death? Health Care Professionals' Narrations on End-of-Life Care," *Death Studies* 38, no. 1 (2014): 20–27; and Linda Ganzini, Elizabeth R. Goy, and Steven K. Dobscha, "Why Oregon Patients Request Assisted Death: Family Members' Views," *Journal of General Internal Medicine* 23, no. 2 (2008): 154–157.

[3] See Ruth Macklin, "Dignity Is a Useless Concept," *BMJ* 327 (2003): 1419–1420; and Stephen Pinker, "The Stupidity of Dignity," *The New Republic*, May 28, 2008, accessed January 10, 2017, https://newrepublic.com/article/64674/the-stupidity-dignity. This choir also includes Alasdair Cochrane, "Undignified Bioethics," *Bioethics* 24, no. 5 (2010): 234–241; Remy Debes, "Dignity's Gauntlet," *Philosophical Perspectives* 23, no. 1 (2009): 45–78; and Ruth Macklin, "Reflections on the Human Dignity Symposium: Is Dignity a Useless Concept?" *Journal of Palliative Care* 20, no. 3 (2004): 212–216.

[4] For recent defenses, see Inmaculada de Melo-Martin, "An Undignified Bioethics: There Is No Method in This Madness," *Bioethics* 26, no. 4 (2012): 224–230; Richard Horton, "Rediscovering Human Dignity," *The Lancet* 364, no. 9439 (2004): 1081–1085; Matthew C. Jordan, "Bioethics and 'Human Dignity,'" *Journal of Medicine and Philosophy* 35, no. 2 (2010): 180–196; Suzy Killmister, "Dignity: Not Such a Useless Concept," *Journal of Medical Ethics* 36, no. 3 (2009): 160–164; David J. Mattson and Susan G. Clark, "Human Dignity in Concept and Practice," *Policy Sciences* 44, no. 4 (2011): 303–319; Thaddeus Metz, "African Conceptions of Human Dignity: Vitality and Community as the Ground of Human Rights," *Human Rights Review* 13, no. 1 (2012): 19–37; Sebastian Muders, "Human Dignity in Bioethics, " *Encyclopedia of Life Sciences* (2017), accessed January 31, 2017, http://www.els.net/WileyCDA/ElsArticle/refId-a0027020.html; and Peter Schaber, "Menschenwürde: Ein für die Medizinethik irrelevanter Begriff?" *Ethik in der Medizin* 24, no. 4 (2012): 297–306.

positions within bioethical debates. There are many articles that try to give a systematic overview of the different theories of human dignity,[5] but much work still needs to be done. Hence the reawakened interest in dignity, which undoubtedly has partly motivated the flood of anthologies[6] and monographs[7] currently on offer.

Although this shows that philosophical thinking about dignity is indeed at its peak, the crucial next step—applying the insights of a general conception of dignity to the ethical issues many societies are currently grappling with—is still underdeveloped. There are a number of book chapters on various applied themes,[8] usually presented within a more general account of what the notion of dignity means for bioethics, literally ranging from human conception to death. In these texts, the authors naturally approach the subject from their specific moral viewpoints and discuss other accounts only from this angle. This makes them less valuable as a rich resource for dignity's applicability in the debate on assisted death.

---

[5] Jane Haddock, "Towards Further Clarification of the Concept 'Dignity,'" *Journal of Advanced Nursing* 24, no. 5 (1996): 924–931; Matti Häyry, "Another Look at Dignity," *Cambridge Quarterly of Healthcare Ethics* 13, no. 1 (2004): 7–14; Nora Jacobson, "Dignity and Health: A Review," *Social Science and Medicine* 64, no. 2 (2006): 292–302; Nora Jacobson, "A Taxonomy of Dignity: A Grounded Theory Study," *BMC International Health and Human Rights* 9, no. 3 (2009), accessed January 10, 2017, https://doi.org/10.1186/1472-698X-9-3; Sebastian Muders, "Natural Good Theories and the Value of Human Dignity," *Cambridge Quarterly of Healthcare Ethics* 25, no. 2 (2016), 239–249; Lennart Nordenfelt, "The Varieties of Dignity," *Health Care Analysis* 12, no. 2 (2004): 83–89; Doris Schroeder, "Dignity: Two Riddles and Four Concepts," *Cambridge Quarterly of Healthcare Ethics* 17, no. 1 (2008): 230–238; and Doris Schroeder, "Dignity: One, Two, Three, Four, Five, Still Counting," *Cambridge Quarterly of Healthcare Ethics* 19, no. 1 (2010): 118–125.

[6] Important examples are Marcus Düwell et al. (eds.), *The Cambridge Handbook of Human Dignity: Interdisciplinary Perspectives* (Cambridge: Cambridge University Press, 2014); Paulus Kaufmann et al. (eds.), *Humiliation, Degradation, Dehumanization: Human Dignity Violated* (Dordrecht: Springer, 2010); Jeff Malpas and Norelle Lickiss (eds.), *Perspectives on Human Dignity* (Dordrecht: Springer, 2007); and Christopher McCrudden (ed.), *Understanding Human Dignity* (Oxford: Oxford University Press, 2014).

[7] Here examples include George Kateb, *Human Dignity* (Cambridge, Mass.: Harvard University Press, 2011); David G. Kirchhoffer, *Human Dignity in Contemporary Bioethics* (Amherst, NY: Teneo Press, 2013); Gilbert Meilaender, *Neither Beast Nor God: The Dignity of the Human Person* (New York: Encounter Books, 2009); Michael Rosen, *Dignity: Its History and Meaning* (Cambridge, Mass.: Harvard University Press, 2012); Peter Schaber, *Instrumentalisierung und Würde* (Paderborn: Mentis, 2010); and Jeremy Waldron, *Dignity, Rank, and Rights* (New York: Oxford University Press, 2012).

[8] See, for instance, Deryck Beyleveld and Roger Brownsword, *Human Dignity in Bioethics and Biolaw* (New York: Oxford University Press, 2001); Stephen Dilley and Nathan J. Palpant (ed.), *Human Dignity in Bioethics: From Worldviews to the Public Square* (New York: Routledge, 2013); Jan C. Joerden, Eric Hilgendorf, and Felix Thiele (eds.), *Menschenwürde und Medizin: Ein interdisziplinäres Handbuch* (Berlin: Duncker & Humblot, 2013); and Christopher Kaczor, *A Defense of Dignity: Creating Life, Destroying Life, and Protecting the Rights of Conscience* (Notre Dame, Ind.: University of Notre Dame Press, 2013).

In summary, although assisted death is still a prominent topic in bio-ethics, the relevance of human dignity for this debate has not yet found the adequate, multifaceted treatment it deserves, namely a treatment that assembles all important perspectives and positions, examines the arguments that may be enhanced by it, and enriches the yet undertheorized role it currently holds in this debate. As the exposition should have made clear, this is a particularly appropriate time for the debate about dignity to be decisively brought to bear on practical ethics.

The aim of this first in-depth examination of the application of human dignity to assisted suicide is threefold. First, the book will enlighten and explain the widely shared intuitions about human dignity, which has a specific usage in the medical context of terminal illness, because opponents as well as supporters of assisted suicide lay claim to that notion. Second, the book will push the debate an important step forward because arguments that are often taken for granted can be more fairly reconsidered once their relationship to dignity has been clarified—for example, arguments from autonomy or self-determination, as well as other arguments that are often neglected as overly theoretical, such as arguments that appeal to the inviolability of (human) life. Third, if one is able to make sense of dignity even within the complex and seemingly confused context of this debate, one will have taken an important step toward a clarification of it in general, which might lead to its application in other contexts as well.

Structure of the Book

This volume is divided into six sections. Section 1 considers the general relevance of the notion of human dignity for the debate on assisted death—whether human dignity is helpful or not to formulate arguments for and against this practice. Here and in the sections that follow, there are two chapters that usually adopt the two main normative standpoints found in the debate—one that is more in favor of assisted death and another that is rather skeptical of it.

In Chapter 2, titled "Human Dignity, Suicide, and Assisting Others to Die," Jeff McMahan is concerned with the question whether dignity can be of any use in the debate on assisted suicide for those who argue against this practice. To this end, he canvasses and critically evaluates various ways of understanding human dignity, including those found in the work of Kant and some contemporary Kantians. In conclusion, he adopts a mainly critical stance of using dignity in an argument against assisted suicide: Nothing that the defenders of a Kantian or capability-based notion of human dignity say is able to justify a general rejection of assisted death.

Whereas McMahan is concerned with employing the notion of human dignity in arguments against the practice of assisted dying, Ralf Stoecker aims at substantiating worries about grounding the right of assisted suicide in dignity. In Chapter 3, "Dignity and the Case in Favor of Assisted Death," he presents two arguments usually brought forward by advocates of the legalization of physician-assisted suicide: According to the first helping people to end their lives is a matter of human dignity because the prohibition to do so interferes with a fundamental liberty to conduct life according to one's own preferences Furthermore, suicide is sometimes an appropriate measure to avoid living an undignified life. Stoecker argues that although the first argument is strong, the second argument is misguided. Hence, from an ethical perspective, society should not legally prohibit physician-assisted suicide. Yet, the person herself should not commit suicide either. In particular, she should not regard such a suicide as a demand of her dignity. *Use*

Following these rather skeptical assessments regarding human dignity's role in the debate on assisted death, the volume turns to more optimistic approaches that seek to include human dignity when making their case for or against this practice. Specifically, Sections 2–5 address the main arguments and lines of reasoning that are linked to human dignity within the debate on assisted dying. These concern the role played by dignity in end-of-life decisions (Section 2) and in cases involving persons with physical and mental disabilities (Section 3) before turning to two arguments that are often used in connection with human dignity: the argument from personal autonomy (Section 4) and the argument from the value of human life (Section 5).

Section 2 situates human dignity within the context in which it is most relevant for debates on assisted suicide—situations near the end of human life, where questions about a "death with dignity" emerge. Here, L. W. Sumner, in his contribution "Dignity through Thick and Thin" (Chapter 4), argues that there is indeed a useful "thick" conception of dignity that can provide some distinctive justification for the pro side of the debate on assisted death: It can be used to give a voice to terminally ill patients who plausibly link some of their welfare-related concerns to human dignity. This way, the conception can be used as a convenient vehicle for collecting many of the good-making features of a good life.

In contrast to this view, in Chapter 5, Robert P. George and Christopher Kazcor argue for the opposing claim: Whereas advocates of euthanasia often use the phrase "death with dignity" to suggest that intentional killing at the end of life secures and protects human dignity, critics of euthanasia insist that intentional killing always violates human dignity, George and Kazcor opt for the latter view. To this end, the authors first distinguish four different senses of the term: dignity as attributed, dignity as intrinsic worth, dignity as flourishing, and dignity as expressing autonomy. They then argue that intentional killing undermines dignity in all four senses applicable to cases of assisted dying.

The contributions in Section 3 are concerned with the role of human dignity in assisted-dying cases that are raised by disability advocates. In particular, they address the worry that public acceptance of assistance in dying, especially beyond "terminal illness" cases, may fatally reinforce the assumption that it is undignified to be severely disabled.

The first contribution, written by David Wasserman (Chapter 6), focuses on the relevance of physical disability for justifying extensions of physician assistance in dying to individuals who are not terminally ill. Wasserman argues that such disabilities, however severe, provide no stronger dignity-based reason than other kinds of loss or misfortune for permitting physician assistance, either as a condition for finding or presuming unbearable suffering or as an independent ground for physician assistance. A law or policy that singled out physical disability, however severe, as supporting a dignity-based claim for physician assistance would be deeply misguided. The state's position should be that there is no inherent indignity in any physical condition or in any degree of physical dependence.

Chapter 7, authored by Rebecca Dresser, deals with some of the distinct issues that surround the relationship of dignity and assisted death for potential or actual dementia patients. In particular, Dresser examines the role of dignity concerns in addressing requests for assisted death as a preemptive measure to avoid a possible future with dementia, requests for assisted death by individuals with mild or moderate dementia, and advance directives requesting assisted death in the event of a later dementia diagnosis or appearance of specific behavioral manifestations of dementia (e.g., apparent inability to recognize family and friends).

Sections 4 and 5 build on the cases discussed in the previous two sections by debating the two most prominent normative phenomena related to assisted suicide that have proven to be highly relevant for both sides of the debate—autonomy and human life. In particular, the chapters in these sections investigate how one might employ them in new and original ways to construct arguments that challenge the boundaries of the "classic" positions for and against assisted suicide.

Beginning with Section 4, which is dedicated to the role of autonomy in the assisted death debate, Sebastian Muders in Chapter 8 follows the current mainstream in analytic ethics, expressing his conviction that dignity is essentially related to respect and self-determination. However, he also believes that these are hardly the only normative components within a promising theory of human dignity that have to be taken into account. He argues that other values, such as the value of human life, must be incorporated as well. To this end, he offers an approach that explicates dignity in terms of specific interpretations of *both* autonomy and life's value, in a way that ascribes a unique normative role to both. This, he claims, does a better job explaining our complex attitudes toward various cases raised in the debate on assisted suicide and euthanasia.

One of the most widely debated conceptions of autonomy that bears a direct connection to human dignity is that of Kant. In Chapter 9, "Dignity and Assisted Dying: What Kant Got Right (and Wrong)," Michael Cholbi's aim is to outline a genuine Kantian understanding of dignity and of its implications for the ethics of assisted dying. Kant's reasoning seems to preclude acts of self-killing, including voluntary assisted dying, that rest on individual self-interest, because a person's interests merely have a price. However, Cholbi argues that a recognizably Kantian view of dignity, although not as permissive as many "liberal" views, can allow assisted dying for agents at least under some circumstances.

The penultimate Section 5 focuses on the argument from the value of life. Similarly to the previous sections, it comprises two texts that take opposing stances toward the role that appeals to human dignity can play in arguments employed for or against assisted dying. Starting from the concept of dignity as referring to the goodness or worth of a life, Luke Gormally argues in Chapter 10 that assisted suicide is rationalised as a benefit on the ground that a life can cease to be worthwhile if what counts as the worth of a life is determined by the choice of the person whose life it is. However, he submits that such a conception is inconsistent with our basic intuitions about justice, while an ontologically based conception of human dignity does fit those intuitions. He claims that this latter conception of dignity stands in the way of any life being judged to be no longer worthwhile, and thus no life is eligible for assisted death.

In Chapter 11, William FitzPatrick argues that, on the contrary, any special value we attribute to human life is derivative from the special value of the human person that this life normally (but not always) subserves. The idea of dignity is relevant to understanding that person-level value, which in turn can be appealed to in support of physician-assisted death in cases in which life is no longer a good for the person. The upshot of his argument is that respect for human dignity is the appropriate focus rather than a more abstract respect for (or valuing of) human life, and the former actually supports the moral appropriateness of physician-assisted death in relevant circumstances because it exhibits proper respect for the (dignity of the) person.

The chapters in Section 6 finally step back slightly from dignity's immediate involvement in the debate on assisted death to examine the relationship between human dignity and rights. This encompasses two questions. The first question is whether dignity can be interpreted as a specific high-graded liberty right, or even qualify as a "fundamental right". A further question is whether dignity might merely assist a pro-choice stance in this debate, instead of being directly relevant to justifying such a stance, by normatively grounding a claim right that generates a duty to provide assisted death.

In Chapter 12, Margaret Battin takes a second look at some ideas she expressed more than thirty-five years ago in her seminal paper "Suicide: A *Fundamental* Human Right?" After examining various attempts to conceive of dignity, Battin remains skeptical about the claim that we actually have a promising conception of dignity that allows us to mark the boundaries of a fundamental right to suicide, and thus between "dignified" and "undignified" suicides. Still, she believes that the possibility remains of developing such a conception, although it may prove to be more difficult than many philosophers might think.

In Chapter 13, Peter Schaber and Holger Baumann argue that human dignity yields an argument in favor of the moral permissibility of assisted suicide. If a person competently requests another person to assist her in dying, she thereby exercises her normative power and makes the act permissible. Denying a person the normative power to make this action permissible means to disrespect her human dignity. They thus argue against views that regard terminating one's own life (by the help of others) as *morally impermissible* for reasons of human dignity. At the same time, however, Baumann and Schaber depart from those views that argue for a *moral duty* to provide assisted suicide by appeal to human dignity. In their view, appeals to human dignity do not yield a duty for the other person to help, nor even reasons in favor of helping. There is, then, no *claim right to assisted suicide* that a person who wants to die might invoke in order to receive help from others.

Earlier versions of roughly half of the chapters in this volume were presented at a workshop on assisted death and human dignity that took place in Zürich, Switzerland on February 5 and 6, 2014. The other half consists of invited contributions. The editor thanks all the authors of this volume for their valuable chapters that will push the debate on assisted dying and human dignity forward.

SECTION 1 | **Human Dignity and the Case of Assisted Death**

CHAPTER 2 | Human Dignity, Suicide, and Assisting Others to Die

JEFF MCMAHAN

Introduction

As Sebastian Muders notes in the introduction to this volume, the notion of human dignity is often invoked on both sides of the debate about the permissibility of assisting others to commit suicide. Some claim that human dignity is what is respected when one assists someone to commit suicide when she rationally wishes to die and her death would not wrongly harm anyone else. Others claim that human dignity is what is violated when one assists someone to commit suicide. The topic of this chapter is whether anything can be said in support of this latter claim. I consider whether a case can be made against the permissibility of assisting someone to commit suicide by appealing to the notion of human dignity. My conclusion is that the best arguments of which I am aware that claim that suicide and assistance in suicide are incompatible with respect for human dignity all fail.

My arguments are almost entirely critical. Before I began to write this essay, my impression was that the notion of human dignity often functions in moral and political writing as a rhetorical substitute for argument. My subsequent research has provided little reason to doubt the accuracy of that initial perception.

Before turning to the arguments, I say a few words about terminology. First, I continue to use the traditional phrase "commit suicide," which can refer both to killing oneself and to allowing oneself to die, despite the pejorative connotations of the word "commit." The phrase is concise and enables one to reduce one's use of gender-specific pronouns, as in "kills herself" or "ends his own life." I hope it will be sufficient just to say explicitly that I intend nothing pejorative when I refer to someone's "committing" suicide.

Second, "assisted suicide" is something that is done by those who commit suicide with assistance from others, not what is done by those who provide the assistance. I assume there is no serious debate about whether it is morally better or morally worse to kill oneself with assistance rather than without it, and thus that discussions that are said to be about "assisted suicide" are generally not concerned with the permissibility of committing suicide with assistance but instead with the permissibility of providing assistance to others who wish to end their own lives.

Human Dignity and Membership in the Human Species

One quite general reason for skepticism about the notion of human dignity is that as it is normally deployed in moral argument, it is speciesist. This is of course immediately suggested by the label but is also confirmed by a survey of the ways in which the notion is defined (when it is defined at all, which is rather seldom) in debates in bioethics and about human rights. In these contexts, human dignity is a property we are supposed to have by virtue of our "common humanity" or merely by virtue of our being human. That is, our dignity supervenes upon our humanity, in the biological sense. Human dignity is thus defined by Francis Fukuyama as "the idea that there is something unique about the human race that entitles every member of the species to a higher moral status than the rest of the natural world."[1] This quotation is characteristic of the literature in which the notion of human dignity is invoked in being unspecific about what precisely it is about being human that endows members of our species with an exalted moral status. This is not surprising, in my view, for as I have argued in previous writings, there is in fact nothing about membership in the human species or in any other biological species that is directly relevant to an individual's moral status.

Those who invoke human dignity to justify certain moral claims often pass over questions about the application of those claims to individuals whose membership in the human species is inconvenient in the context. I recall, for example, a presentation by Martha Nussbaum at a conference on cognitive disability in 2008 in which she argued that "showing equal

---

[1] Francis Fukuyama, *Our Posthuman Future: Consequences of the Biotechnology Revolution* (New York: Farrar, Strauss, and Giroux, 2002), 149.

respect for the dignity of citizens with cognitive disabilities requires giving them an equal right to vote, to serve on juries, and so forth." To deny even the most profoundly or radically cognitively impaired adults these legal rights of equal citizenship is, she argued, an offense against their human dignity, which they share equally with other human beings. Thus, radically cognitively impaired adults who are incapable of having thoughts about politics or criminal justice should be assigned surrogates who could act on their behalf in voting and serving on juries.[2] During the discussion, I asked whether her claims extended as well to children, newborn infants, including anencephalic infants, and even fetuses. My recollection (admittedly fallible) is that she was unprepared to endorse the necessity of providing surrogates to vote on behalf of fetuses and infants but did not offer an explanation of why it is an offense against human dignity to deny the right to vote to an adult with psychological capacities no higher than those of an infant but not to deny the same right to an infant.

Elsewhere in her work, Nussbaum argues that the possession of various "capabilities" is necessary for a human being to have "a life worthy of human dignity." Here, dignity seems to be a certain status we have by virtue of being human that entitles us to certain forms of treatment, including being provided with the capabilities or with the conditions for having them. Having the capabilities, moreover, seems to be *constitutive* of what it is to have a life that is *worthy* of human dignity—that is, worthy of someone who has human dignity. Thus, she says, "a life without a sufficient level of each of these entitlements is a life so reduced that it is not compatible with human dignity."[3]

Yet among the 10 "central human capabilities" are being able to form a conception of the good and having the bases of self-respect. It is quite impossible for radically cognitively impaired human beings to have these capabilities when, like infants and most nonhuman animals, they lack the capacity for self-consciousness. It seems to follow that their lives are incompatible with human dignity and cannot be made compatible with it, at least until some form of cognitive enhancement is developed that could cause them to develop the capacity for self-consciousness. Yet Nussbaum's claims about the rights of citizenship presuppose that these human beings do have human dignity. Thus, although they have human dignity, they

---

[2] Nussbaum's talk was later published as "The Capabilities of People with Cognitive Disabilities," *Metaphilosophy* 40, no. 3–4 (2009): 331–351. The quotation in the text is from p. 333.
[3] Martha Craven Nussbaum, *Frontiers of Justice: Disability, Nationality, Species Membership* (Cambridge, Mass.: Belknap, 2007), 278–279.

also have lives that cannot be made compatible with human dignity. It is unclear what conclusion one should draw from this.

Certainly Nussbaum would have to reject the view of David Velleman, who is among those who believe that human dignity forbids bringing about people's deaths just so that they can avoid a future life in which the bad elements, such as suffering, would outweigh the good. This is because Velleman does accept the permissibility of bringing about the death of a person when his life would otherwise become incompatible with or "offend against" his human dignity. "When a person cannot sustain both life and dignity," Velleman writes, "his death may indeed be morally justified. One is sometimes permitted, even obligated, to destroy objects of dignity if they would otherwise deteriorate in ways that would offend against that value."[4] So Nussbaum's view implies that the life of a human being who lacks the capacity to form a conception of the good is incompatible with human dignity. And Velleman holds that it may be obligatory to destroy a human being whose life offends against, and is thus incompatible with, human dignity. The combination of these views seems to entail that it can be permissible, or even obligatory, to put radically cognitively impaired human beings to death to prevent their lives from continuing to undermine their human dignity.

Of course, neither would accept such an absurd and repugnant claim. The problem results from their having quite different understandings of the nature and moral significance of human dignity—a problem that seems pervasive in the literature in which the notion of human dignity is conscripted to do substantive moral work. Although the notion of human dignity is ubiquitous in writing on issues in bioethics and on the foundations of human rights, it is a highly protean term. As I remarked previously, its function often seems more rhetorical than substantive.

Among the questions that have to be answered are the following: What does "human dignity" mean or refer to? Do you and I really have it? If so, what properties or capacities do we share that are the basis of our having it? That is, on which natural properties does human dignity supervene? Do all human beings have these properties while no nonhuman animals do? If we do have human dignity, does that make it impermissible to commit suicide? Does it likewise make it impermissible to assist someone to commit suicide? That is, are suicide, assisting suicide, and euthanasia incompatible with respect for human dignity?

---

[4] J. David Velleman, "A Right of Self-Termination?", *Ethics* 109 (1999): 606–628, 617.

Character and Rank

In an article from a few years ago, Charles Beitz surveys various ways in which the notion of human dignity has figured in philosophical and legal writing, particularly about human rights.[5] Following Michael Rosen, he distinguishes four "strands" of thought about the nature of dignity in the history of philosophical and legal thought. One of these strands, according to which dignity is a kind of value, is the subject of the next section. Of the other three, two are irrelevant to the debate about helping people to commit suicide—namely, the strand that understands dignity as a virtue, or manner of character, and that which understands it as deservingness of respect on account of that virtue or character. One reason these are irrelevant for our purposes is that they are concerned with *personal* dignity rather than *human* dignity; thus, these forms of dignity may be possessed by some persons but not others. They are not, in other words, universal among human beings. Moreover, although the Stoics thought that dignity in this sense might *require* suicide in certain circumstances, no one supposes that it is wrong to assist a person to commit suicide because she is dignified in manner or character but permissible to assist someone who is undignified in these ways.

A third strand that is distinguished by Rosen and Beitz may also seem irrelevant to the permissibility of suicide and assisting others to commit suicide. This is the use of dignity to refer to high social *rank*. The philosopher who has done most to elucidate the notion of human dignity by reference to this tradition of thought is Jeremy Waldron, who writes that "the modern notion of *human* dignity involves an upwards equalization of rank, so that we now try to accord to every human being something of the dignity, rank, and expectation of respect that was formerly accorded to nobility."[6] On this basis, he claims that "we are all chiefs. . . . We all stand proud, and . . . look up to each other from a position of upright equality."[7]

Among the various obstacles to importing this understanding of human dignity into discussions of the permissibility of suicide and of assisting others to commit suicide is that this form of dignity seems to be socially conferred rather than intrinsic. Whether we have dignity in this sense is a matter of social organization and the attitudes of others. And it seems that

---

[5] Charles R. Beitz, "Human Dignity in the Theory of Human Rights: Nothing But a Phrase?" *Philosophy and Public Affairs* 41 (2013): 259–290.
[6] Quoted in Beitz, "Human Dignity in the Theory of Human Rights," 283.
[7] Beitz, "Human Dignity in the Theory of Human Rights," 284.

whether a person has been accorded the highest social standing is irrelevant to whether it is permissible for her to commit suicide or for others to assist her to commit suicide.

Nor is this understanding of dignity applicable to all human beings. No fetus or infant can be a chief or stand proud. An infant can, of course, look up to others, but not, even figuratively, from a position of upright equality. Thus, despite Waldron's claim that the idea of equality of rank is a notion of "*human* dignity," it is, at most, a notion of *adult* human dignity. And it is probably not even that, as it is difficult even to understand what would be involved in according to radically cognitively impaired adults "the dignity, rank, and expectation of respect that was formerly accorded to nobility."

In an effort to extract some implications for human rights from the notion of dignity identified by Waldron, Beitz observes that one important way in which nobles, during the age of nobility, were different from others is that they had a much greater capacity for self-direction. He then suggests that

> if human dignity is an extension of the noble's special status to all then perhaps we should understand the package of entitlements that defines "human" status as those necessary to enable and protect the effective exercise of the capacity for self-direction by everyone.

We might then understand "human dignity as the status of a self-directing agent."[8]

Quite apart from the recurrent problem that many human beings lack the capacities, such as the capacity for self-direction, that are associated with various conceptions of dignity, there is reason to doubt whether what Beitz suggests is even possible. For it is arguable that it was essential to the nobles' exceptional capacity for self-direction that they had a greater capacity to direct the lives of *others*—not just greater than that of their non-noble contemporaries but also greater than that possessed by most people now who enjoy the highest level of social recognition. If so, the vision of everyone having the expectation of respect that nobles enjoyed is unrealistic. We cannot all be kings, as there cannot be kings without subjects.

But even if Beitz's suggestion were feasible, it would offer no basis for a moral objection to suicide or to assisting someone to commit suicide. On

---

[8] Beitz, "Human Dignity in the Theory of Human Rights," 286.

the contrary, understanding our capacity for self-direction as fundamental to our moral status suggests instead that suicide should come within the scope of our entitlement to act on our capacity for self-direction.

Another idea one frequently finds in contemporary discussions (for example, in the work of Jürgen Habermas and Avishai Margalit) is that human dignity is that which is violated when a person is unjustly humiliated. Yet again, however, this notion provides no basis for an objection to suicide or to assisting others to commit suicide. One does not necessarily humiliate oneself by committing suicide (which one may, as the Stoics showed, do with great dignity of manner). Nor does one necessarily humiliate another person, or oneself, by helping her to commit suicide. On the contrary, there are circumstances in which suicide is the only means of avoiding humiliation, either at the hands of human tormenters or because of the inevitability of mental or physical deterioration.

Kantian Arguments

Kant's Conception of Human Dignity

The philosophical tradition to which contemporary thought about human dignity is most indebted is that deriving from the work of Immanuel Kant. In his *Groundwork of the Metaphysics of Morals*, Kant writes that dignity is "an inner worth," an "unconditional, incomparable worth, for which the word *respect* alone makes a befitting expression of the estimation a rational being is to give it." He contrasts dignity with *price*, which "can be replaced with something else, as its *equivalent.*" Dignity, he observes, is "infinitely above any price, with which it cannot be balanced or compared at all." He also writes that "*autonomy* is . . . the ground of the dignity of a human and of every rational nature."[9]

These passages have been interpreted by most contemporary philosophers who have studied Kant's moral philosophy as stating a doctrine of human dignity according to which all human beings have an inherent value or worth that cannot be outweighed by, or even weighed against, other values. Although Kant says that "autonomy" is the ground of dignity in human beings, many Kantian philosophers have used the other phrase that appears in this quotation, "rational nature," to refer to that which is

---

[9] Immanuel Kant, *Groundwork of the Metaphysics of Morals*, edited by Mary Gregor and Jens Timmermann, revised edition (Cambridge: Cambridge University Press, 2012), 4:435 and 4:436; emphases in original.

the basis of human dignity. Other scholars note that Kant sometimes refers to that which grounds our dignity as our "humanity" or "humanity in our person." Some believe that these terms are roughly synonymous with "rational capacity" or "rational nature." This is supported by Kant's writing, at one point, that "*a rational nature exists as an end in itself*" and then, a few lines later, referring to "humanity, *as an end it itself.*"[10] But some, including Derek Parfit, believe that "humanity" refers "not to our rationality, but either to our capacity for acting morally and having a good will, or to ourselves as what Kant calls *noumenal* beings."[11] Parfit may, however, believe the same about "rational nature."

It is not clear how substantively significant these interpretive issues are. There are, however, some disagreements among scholars about Kant's understanding of dignity that are highly relevant to understanding the implications of Kant's philosophy for the morality of suicide and assistance in suicide. Oliver Sensen, for example, has argued that Kant does not understand dignity in anything like the way I have just outlined. On the basis of meticulous attention to Kant's texts, and issues of consistency among various relevant passages, he contends that Kant in fact has no conception of a value inherent in human beings that grounds a requirement to respect them, that the requirement to respect them is instead a direct command of reason, and that Kant believes that human beings have dignity because they must be respected—*not* that they must be respected because they have dignity. According to Sensen, Kant's actual conception of dignity is a compound of elements of the conceptions reviewed in the preceding section. On his understanding of Kant's view, to have dignity is to have an elevated rank or status and also, perhaps, to have a character worthy of that rank or appropriate for those of that rank.[12]

I will not attempt to resolve or even to contribute to these exegetical debates. As Sensen observes, the conception of dignity that he attributes to Kant is traceable to the Stoics, and in particular to Cicero's ascription of *dignitas* to all human beings because of their elevated place in nature.[13] Rather than challenging the permissibility of suicide and assistance in suicide, the Stoic understanding of human dignity is that our status as rational beings requires us to choose, if possible, when and how we are to die. Kant apparently had some admiration for this view. Despite his explicit and

[10] Kant, *Groundwork of the Metaphysics of Morals*, 4:429; emphases in original.

[11] Derek Parfit, *On What Matters, Volume One* (Oxford: Oxford University Press, 2011), 242.

[12] Oliver Sensen, *Kant on Human Dignity* (Berlin: De Gruyter, 2011).

[13] Sensen, *Kant on Human Dignity*, 155–157.

repeated denunciations of suicide, he is reported to have said in a lecture that "in the Stoic's principle concerning suicide there lay much sublimity of soul: that we may depart from life as we leave a smoky room."[14] (He is referring here to the following words of Epictetus: "Has it smoked in the chamber? If the smoke is moderate, I will stay; if it is excessive, I go out: For you must always remember . . . that the door is open."[15])

The Lexical Priority Argument

Because Sensen's interpretation of Kant's conception of dignity provides no support for the view that suicide and assistance in suicide are impermissible, I will not consider it further. My concern, as I have stated, is with views that understand human dignity in ways that challenge the permissibility of suicide. The more common interpretation of Kant's conception of human dignity, according to which dignity is a value inherent in human beings that is grounded in their rational nature, is widely held to be a view of this sort.

As mentioned previously, Kant states that dignity is an "incomparable worth" that "cannot be balanced or compared at all" with anything of price—which means, in effect, anything else of value. According to various distinguished interpreters of Kant, the reason why this is so is that our dignity is grounded in or supervenes upon our rational nature, which is, through our rationally willing our ends, the source of all value other than its own.[16] And that which is the source of value, or at least of all value that has a price, must have value of a different kind: namely, unconditional value that cannot be exchanged with other, lesser values. Thus it is that rational nature has dignity, and that we have dignity by virtue of our rational nature.

From this, some contemporary Kantians infer the impermissibility of suicide, or at least suicide committed for reasons other than the avoidance of the degradation of rational nature. David Velleman, for example, begins

---

[14] Immanuel Kant, *Lectures on Ethics*, edited by Peter Heath and J. B. Schneewind (Cambridge: Cambridge University Press, 2001), 27:628.

[15] Epictetus, *Discourses of Epictetus*, translated by George Long (New York: Appleton, 1904), 70.

[16] For example, Christine Korsgaard, *The Sources of Normativity* (Cambridge: Cambridge University Press, 1996); Christine Korsgaard, *Creating the Kingdom of Ends* (Cambridge: Cambridge University Press, 1996); and Alison Hills, "Rational Nature as the Source of Value," *Kantian Review* 10 (2005): 60–81. For a related view, see Allen Wood, *Kant's Ethical Thought* (Cambridge: Cambridge University Press, 1999). For forceful criticism, see William J. FitzPatrick, "The Practical Turn in Ethical Theory: Korsgaard's Constructivism, Realism, and the Nature of Normativity," *Ethics* 115 (2005): 651–691, esp. sections IV and V.

with the widely accepted claims that Kant "attributes dignity to all persons in virtue of their rational nature" and that "what morality requires of us, according to Kant, is that we respect the dignity of persons."[17] He goes on to quote Kant's formula of humanity from the *Groundwork*, which asserts that the object of respect "must . . . be conceived . . . as an end against which we should never act, and consequently as one which in all our willing we must never rate *merely* as a means."[18] He then comments that "the violation" that respect must motivate us not to commit "can be conceived as that of using the object as a mere means to other ends."[19] And precisely this violation occurs, he claims, when a person commits suicide to avoid pain, suffering, or further life that would be, for whatever other reason, intrinsically bad: "To destroy something just because it no longer does one more good than harm is to treat it as an instrument of one's interests."[20] Thus, to destroy oneself as a means of avoiding harm is to use an entity that has dignity as an instrument in the service of a lesser value, one that has mere price and hence cannot outweigh, or even weigh against, the literally incomparable worth of dignity. Respect for dignity, in other words, always has lexical priority over the protection or promotion of well-being. And to "trad[e] one's person in exchange for . . . relief from harm" is a violation of the requirement of respect for human dignity.[21] We can refer to this form of objection to suicide and assistance in suicide as the *lexical priority argument*.

In these quoted passages, Velleman emphasizes the claim that one who commits suicide to avoid an intrinsically bad life *uses* herself (her person, her rational nature, her humanity, etc.) *instrumentally* in the achievement of her end. Both common-sense morality and many contemporary philosophers accept that this mode of agency can be specially morally objectionable. This may be seen in the contrast between two versions of the familiar case of a runaway trolley. In one version, a bystander can divert a trolley that will otherwise kill five people so that it will instead kill only one person on a different track. In this version, the person killed is not used as a means of saving the five but is killed as a side effect of the diversion of the trolley away from them. In the second version, however,

---

[17] Velleman, "A Right of Self-Termination?", 611.

[18] Velleman here quotes from Immanuel Kant, *Groundwork of the Metaphysics of Morals*, translated by H. J. Paton (New York: Harper and Row, 1964), 4:437. The quotation is in J. David Velleman, "Love as a Moral Emotion," *Ethics* 109 (1999): 338–374, 359.

[19] Velleman, "Love as a Moral Emotion," 360.

[20] Velleman, "A Right of Self-Termination?", 624.

[21] Velleman, "A Right of Self-Termination?", 614.

an innocent bystander is killed by being maneuvered into the path of the trolley to serve as a shield of the five. Most people believe that there is a significant moral difference between the two versions, and many believe that the killing in the second version is especially objectionable because it involves harmfully *using* a person as an instrument in the service of the interests of others.

But to kill oneself as a means of avoiding a harmful future life involves a quite different mode of agency. In the second trolley case, the presence of the innocent bystander is necessary for the saving of the five. In general, an instrument must be present to be used. Yet one who commits suicide as a means of avoiding harm does not require her own presence so that she can use herself. Rather, her presence is part of the problem and in the circumstances is presumably the only part of the problem over which she can exert control (for if she could eliminate the threatened harm rather than the potential victim, she would do so).

Warren Quinn distinguishes the form of agency in this case, which he calls "eliminative agency," from that in the second trolley case, which he calls "opportunistic agency," remarking that it is natural to suppose that the latter is normally more objectionable than the former.[22] Both involve acting with an intention to affect an individual as a means. The difference is that in opportunistic agency one uses someone's presence as an opportunity to gain a benefit, whereas in eliminative agency one seeks only to eliminate a threat or problem that someone poses.

Although eliminative agency involves intending to affect someone as a means, the eliminative harming of an innocent person is generally regarded, perhaps surprisingly, as *less* morally problematic than inflicting the same harm on the same innocent person as a foreseen but unintended side effect. Suppose, for example, that one's life is threatened by a person who is wholly lacking in responsibility for the threat he poses. We might imagine, as in one familiar example, that his body has been hurled in one's direction. One can save one's life, but only in one of two ways. One can either kill the nonresponsible threatener or deflect him in a way that will be harmless to him but will kill an innocent bystander as a side effect. If asked about this choice, most people, I think, would say that one ought to kill the threatener rather than the bystander. This is because most people, I think, believe that it would be permissible to kill the threatener, whereas

---

[22] Warren Quinn, "Actions, Intentions, and Consequences: The Doctrine of Double Effect," *Philosophy and Public Affairs* 18 (1989): 334–351, 344.

many believe that it would be impermissible to kill the bystander, even if killing the threatener were not an option.

Killing oneself, or allowing oneself to die, as a means of avoiding a harmful future is thus at least two steps removed from harmful opportunistic agency, which is the form of agency that common-sense morality and many moral philosophers regard as particularly objectionable. For ending one's life in these circumstances is neither harmful nor opportunistic. It benefits the only person who is directly affected and is at most eliminative. I say "at most" because it is in fact only a borderline instance even of eliminative agency. In core cases of eliminative agency, the person who is intentionally affected by the agent's action is herself the source of a threat to or problem for the agent. But a person who commits suicide to avoid a harmful future is not the source of the potential harm. She avoids harm not by eliminating a threat someone poses but, rather, by eliminating the potential victim.

Nothing I have said thus far refutes the lexical priority argument. The foregoing comments do, however, suggest that the argument should be refocused or perhaps just stated differently. For Velleman's references to using people and treating them as instruments are inessential to the argument and indeed are distractions from the central point, which is that because our rational nature is, according to Kant, the source of all values that have price, it has dignity, so that respect for rational nature has lexical priority over all such lower values. The destruction of rational nature, whether as an intended effect or as a foreseen but unintended effect, is a violation of the requirement of respect for human dignity, except in those rare instances in which the destruction of rational nature is required by respect for rational nature itself.[23] Thus, because suicide involves the destruction of one's rational nature, it cannot be justified by the aim or end of avoiding harm, no matter how great the harm would be. This is true whether one uses oneself opportunistically as a means of preventing harm, prevents the harm by preemptively eliminating the potential victim, or destroys one's rational nature only as a side effect of the prevention of harm.

Even when stated this way, however, the lexical priority argument seems to me highly implausible. In part this is because of the metaethics it presupposes. I cannot believe that we, through our rational willing, create all value other than our own. There is, moreover, as the foregoing

---

[23] See Velleman, "A Right of Self-Termination?", 617.

autobiographical detail indicates, a curious tension within Kantian meta-ethics. It is anti-realist about all value with price but realist about the dignity of rational nature.

I cannot, of course, offer a defense of moral realism here (or indeed anywhere else).[24] There are, however, various other objections to the lexical priority argument that I can present here. The first is, perhaps, less an objection than an observation about the restricted scope of the argument. It is a crucial premise that we have dignity because, through our rational willing of our ends, we are the sources of value in the world. But not all human beings are included within this "we," for not all human beings are capable of rationally willing ends for themselves. Not all human beings, in other words, have rational nature, and therefore not all human beings have dignity.

Perhaps Kant believed that all human beings have rational nature in the noumenal realm or that their noumenal selves have rational nature even if their phenomenal selves do not (although it seems a mystery not only how one could know this but also how one could know that animals lack such well-endowed noumenal selves). Speaking for myself, I can make no sense of the suggestion that a human fetus has libertarian free will and the capacity for pure practical reason in its noumenal or intelligible form. To his credit, Velleman parts with Kant on this issue, noting that what "morality must regard as sacrosanct . . . is not the human organism but the person, and a fetus may embody one but not the other."[25] What this means, however, is that the lexical priority argument does not rule out euthanasia in the case of fetuses, newborn infants, or even adults whose cognitive impairments (most obviously when they are congenital but perhaps also when they are acquired) render them incapable of rationally setting ends for themselves.

The most important objections to the lexical priority argument concern its implications for various forms of action. I have argued elsewhere, for example, that if the argument is understood to rule out not just suicide and assistance in suicide but also such acts as impairing a person's rational capacities, subverting a person's rational capacities through torture, enslaving someone, and consenting to become a slave, it will also imply the impermissibility of ingesting a stupefying analgesic or accepting anesthesia as a means of avoiding suffering, as well as administering

---

[24] There are, of course, many such defenses on offer. The most influential is in Derek Parfit, *On What Matters, Volume Two* (Oxford: Oxford University Press, 2011).

[25] Velleman, "A Right of Self-Termination?", 616.

such therapies to others.[26] I will not rehearse those arguments here but will note some other implications that are at least equally absurd.

According to Kant, human dignity cannot be forfeited through wrong-doing.[27] Suppose that a person will culpably and without justification cause a large number of people to suffer, or to become paralyzed, unless he is killed. The harms that he threatens to cause would neither destroy nor even impair the victims' rational natures. They would affect the victims' well-being, but that is a matter of price. Despite his imminent and egregious wrongdoing, the threatener retains his human dignity, and killing him would destroy his rational nature. Killing him as a means of protecting values that have only price would therefore be a violation of the requirement of respect for his human dignity. It seems to follow that neither the victims nor third parties may permissibly kill him in defense of his intended victims.

Kant, or perhaps contemporary Kantians, might formulate universalizable maxims intended to show that both self-defense and other-defense would in this case not only be permissible but also be duties. (Unlike some other moral philosophers, Kant insists that there are duties to the self, such as the duty not to kill oneself. He can therefore recognize a self-regarding duty of self-defense.) But the problem is to explain how the recognition of such duties could be consistent with the view that respect for human dignity is lexically prior to the protection of well-being.

The problem of justifying defensive killing may be more tractable in war than in cases of individual self-defense because soldiers tend to pose lethal threats, which are threats to rational nature. But there are other problems that are well illustrated by examples drawn from war. One such example has long been seen as a challenge to the view that suicide is immoral—namely, the example of the soldier who flings himself on a grenade as a means of saving his comrades. Traditional attempts to show that self-sacrificial action of this sort is not within the scope of the prohibition of suicide—for example, because the soldier does not intend his own death and so does not commit suicide at all—tend to be undermined by consideration of the parallel case in which the soldier throws not himself

---

[26] Jeff McMahan, *The Ethics of Killing: Problems at the Margins of Life* (New York: Oxford University Press, 2002), 480–481.

[27] Parfit writes that "on Kant's view, as Wood and Herman claim, 'even the worst human beings have dignity,' and a person whose will is good 'is of no greater value' than someone with an ordinary or bad will" (*On What Matters, Volume One*, 240). His references are to Wood, *Kant's Ethical Thought*, 133; and to Barbara Herman, *The Practice of Moral Judgment* (Cambridge, Mass.: Harvard University Press, 1993), 238.

but, rather, another soldier on the grenade; for, by parity of reasoning, if the soldier does not intend the death of the one he throws on the grenade, he cannot be guilty of murder. But whether the soldier commits suicide by covering the grenade is not the relevant issue for the lexical priority argument. The problem is, rather, that if the explosion of the grenade would not kill any of the soldier's comrades but would grievously wound them (for example, by tearing the limbs off of a great many of them), his shielding them from these harms would destroy his rational nature but would protect only values of price. In these conditions, his self-sacrificial action would not be noble but immoral.

Similarly, suppose that resources in the health care system are limited and that doctors can either save one person's life or prevent hundreds of people from becoming quadriplegic. If the protection of rational nature has lexical priority over the prevention of any amount of harm that is merely a matter of price, then doctors ought to save the one person's life rather than prevent any number of people from becoming paralyzed.

Finally, there is the problem of risking one's life. Kant himself, after stating the formula of humanity and explaining why it prohibits suicide as a means of avoiding harm, explicitly passes over one question about risk. He writes, in a parenthesis, that "I must here pass over the closer determination of this principle, needed to avoid any misunderstanding, e.g., of amputating limbs to preserve myself, of putting my life in danger to preserve my life, etc.; that belongs to actual moral science."[28]

The challenge to the lexical priority argument, however, comes not from the possibility of risking one's life as a means of saving one's life, which is to risk one's rational nature for the sake of rational nature, but from the possibility of risking one's life in the pursuit of goods with prices, which we do continually. When one drives to the store to buy ice cream, one exposes oneself to a greater risk of death than one would have been under had one stayed at home. But if one's rational nature has lexical priority over happiness, as Kant seems to say it has and some contemporary Kantians say it has, then it must be impermissible to risk the destruction of one's rational nature for the sake of one's happiness. Just as the notion of lexical priority implies that the value or worth of one's rational nature cannot be outweighed by any amount of happiness, so it also implies that there is no risk to one's rational nature that is sufficiently small that it can be outweighed by some sufficiently large probability of some amount of

---

[28] Kant, *Groundwork*, 4:429.

happiness. Driving to buy ice cream, rather than staying at home and doing without, is therefore a violation of respect for human dignity. I take this to be a *reductio ad absurdum* of the lexical priority argument.

The Mere Means Argument

Kant does not explicitly state or endorse the lexical priority argument. When he discusses suicide in the *Groundwork*, he argues that its impermissibility is implied by two of the formulas of the Categorical Imperative. The argument based on the formula of the universal law of nature does not directly appeal to the notion of dignity and seems to me wholly implausible, even in Kant's own terms.[29] For these reasons, I will not discuss it here.

The important argument for our purposes is that which is based on the formula of humanity. That formulation of the Categorical Imperative is:

> So act that you use humanity, in your own person as well as in the person of any other, always at the same time as an end, never merely as a means.

After stating this principle, he immediately draws out what he takes to be its implications for the permissibility of suicide:

> According to the concept of necessary duty to oneself, someone who is contemplating self-murder will ask himself whether his action can be consistent with the idea of humanity, *as an end in itself*. If to escape from a troublesome condition he destroys himself, he makes use of a person, merely as *a means*, to preserve a bearable condition up to the end of life. But a human being is not a thing, hence not something that can be used *merely* as a means, but must in all his actions always be considered as an end in itself. Thus the human being in my own person is not at my disposal, so as to maim, to corrupt, or to kill him.[30]

It is evident from this passage that in articulating the lexical priority argument by reference to the notion of *using as a means* (that is, opportunistic agency), Velleman is being faithful to Kant's own language. But, as we have seen, a person who kills herself to avoid a future that would be intrinsically bad for her does not *use* herself as an *instrument* in the service of

---

[29] Kant, *Groundwork*, 4:422.
[30] Kant, *Groundwork*, 4:429; emphases in original.

her well-being. She does, however, kill herself *as a means* of avoiding misery or suffering. The relevant question for Kant, therefore, is whether, in killing herself as a means, she in fact treats herself *merely* as a means or, as Kant says, as a mere *thing*.

It seems obvious that she does not. Rather, she commits suicide *for her own sake*. Her reason for killing herself testifies to her conviction that she matters in her own right, or for her own sake—that is, that she is an end in herself rather than a mere means.

In a book I published some years ago, I argued that the same is true when a person assists another to commit suicide or kills him at his own request with the intention of benefiting him. There I wrote that, according to Kant,

> it may be permissible to treat a person instrumentally provided that what one does is compatible with his status as an end. This should in fact be obvious, for, as others have pointed out, we regularly treat people instrumentally without denying their worth. We do this when we use them for our purposes but in ways that are compatible with the acknowledgement that they matter in themselves just as we ourselves do—that is, in ways that are respectful of their good, their autonomous will, and their status as rational beings. . . . [So], even if to kill a person when this is both what is best for him and what he autonomously desires is to treat him instrumentally in the service of his good, it is also at the same time to treat him as an end. We defer to his will and secure his good precisely because we recognize that he matters in himself. If we kill him precisely in order to promote his good in accordance with his autonomous desire, it is hard to see how we could be treating him *merely* as a means, as if he did not matter in himself.[31]

These points still seem to me essentially correct. When a person commits suicide to avoid a future life that would be intrinsically bad for her, or when another person assists her to do so for the same reason, neither uses her instrumentally and neither treats her as a mere means. Both treat her as a being who matters for her own sake—that is, as an end in herself. It seems to me, therefore, that Kant's appeals to human dignity provide no better grounds for objecting to the permissibility of suicide and assistance in suicide than the arguments considered in earlier sections.[32]

---

[31] McMahan, *The Ethics of Killing*, 483–484.

[32] I am greatly indebted to Bernhard Koch for discussions of Kant's moral philosophy and to Derek Parfit for comments on an earlier draft of this chapter.

CHAPTER 3 | Dignity and the Case in Favor
of Assisted Suicide

RALF STOECKER

IN ETHICAL DEBATES on the legitimacy of assisted suicide (and other variants of voluntary euthanasia), recourse to human dignity usually is employed on both sides, by opponents as well as advocates. Opponents typically connect a person's dignity with the value of life, whereas advocates see it as matter of respect for human dignity that people get help in ending their lives. In this chapter, I concentrate on the second side—that is, I merely consider whether human dignity speaks in favor of assisted suicide.

That assisted suicide might secure human dignity is a very popular idea. One of the most prominent organizations for assisted suicide in Europe is called "Dignitas"; American laws regulating assisted suicide are called "Death with Dignity Acts" (e.g., the "Washington Death with Dignity Act"); and numerous academic defenders of assisted suicide use the phrase "death with dignity" as a title or starting point for their argumentation. Apparently, the concept of dignity suits the intuitions very well that motivate people to fight for the legalization of physician-assisted death.

Why should we consider a legal prohibition of assisted suicide as a threat to human dignity? There are two different answers to this question: (1) because the prohibition interferes with a fundamental liberty to conduct life according to one's own preferences and any restriction of this liberty violates one's dignity and (2) because sometimes suicide is an appropriate measure to avoid living an undignified life. Ethical debates usually focus on the first answer, defending the individual right to die against external restrictions and limitations. I take it, however, that many public activists and supporters are more concerned with the latter argument. They defend a right to death with dignity, not because it is part of their general right of self-determination but, rather, because they are afraid that without this right they might be forced into leading an undignified life for the last span of their existence.

In this chapter, I concentrate on the second line of argument. Only at the very end do I pick up the first line, too, taking it almost for granted that legal prohibitions of assisted suicide would indeed violate our right to self-determination. However, what I want to show is that contrary to the second line of argument, dignity does not provide us with good reasons to exercise our right to end our lives at will. Quite the contrary, by assuming that in end-of-life situations it is sometimes more dignified to commit suicide than to continue living, we express a morally dubious attitude of contempt to other people. In short, although we have a right to commit suicide and to receive help in killing ourselves, we should better not do so; in particular, we should not see it as a demand of our dignity.

The idea that ending one's life could help secure one's dignity is not surprising, given the long history of committing suicide on the grounds of dignity. Here are two ancient stories. First, near the end of the Trojan War, after Achilles' death, Ulysses and Ajax, two of the mightiest Greek heroes, had a fight about Achilles' weapons. Ulysses won; Ajax was so mad about his defeat that his consciousness became clouded and he killed a goat, which he mistook for Ulysses. Then, when he woke up and realized how he had made a fool of himself by slaughtering the goat, he felt so embarrassed that he immediately stabbed himself to death with his sword. Second, a few hundred years before Christ, a Roman prince raped Lucretia, wife of a consul. The victim, after telling her husband about the insult, killed herself with a dagger in order to wipe out the shame.

As the previous examples illustrate, suicide traditionally has been a well-established measure for protecting or restoring one's dignity. This was confirmed in ancient philosophy. Seneca praised the possibility of committing suicide as a ready means for securing a decent life: "The best thing which eternal law ever ordained was that it allowed to us one entrance into life, but many exits," he wrote, since "it is not important whether we die faster or slower, but whether we die decently or wretchedly" (Seneca, *Letters to Lucilius 70*, author's translation). Evidently, for Ajax and Lucretia, the continuation of their lives would have amounted to leading a wretched life, whereas killing themselves secured their dignity.

The idea that the availability of suicide provides us with a mighty instrument for safeguarding our dignity continued to play an important role in the intellectual assessment of suicide throughout history and does so today. Here are three examples that are relatively recent. In July 1944, General Henning von Tresckow, one of the conspirers against Hitler, blew himself up with a grenade in order to avoid being arrested, tortured, and dishonored. In December 2012, Jacintha Saldanha, a nurse in a London hospital, took her life because she felt deeply embarrassed and humiliated after falling for a prank call from two Australian radio presenters who were pretending to be Prince Charles and the Queen to obtain medical information about Princess Kate. Finally, in January 2016, Geeta, a 40-year-old Indian worker and mother of three children, committed suicide after having been raped by a young man from her neighborhood who had taken a video of his deed and posted it on a popular instant messenger. Evidently, like the nurse, she killed herself in order to avoid living in shame.

The previous examples show that we are still familiar with the idea of persons committing suicide for the sake of dignity. Consequently, we should have no principled problems with other people helping these agents in killing themselves. The soldier, for example, who provided von Tresckow with the grenade was helping him in supporting his dignity and hence presumably did the right thing. The same would have been true if the assistance had not come from a fellow soldier but, rather, from a physical doctor and if the doctor had provided assistance not with a grenade but with the prescription of a lethal drug. A physician's assistance in suicide can therefore be a laudable act of saving a person's dignity.

However, if this is agreed, then we have at least a presumption in favor of the legalization and even institutionalization of physician-assisted suicide as a means for securing the dignity of our fellow citizens. This is the upshot of the second line of argument mentioned previously: Why not have a "Death with Dignity Act" everywhere that allows people to obtain medical support if they decide to strengthen their dignity by ending their lives?

Although my consideration is in the line of the second argument, advocates of the legitimization of physician-assisted suicide might believe that it is proving far too much. After all, the ethical debate is usually not concerned with examples such as resistance fighters and assaulted women. Instead, it is focused on a very special group of suicides, namely suicides by severely ill people who are about to die anyhow or by people who suffer from strongly impairing diseases.[1]

---

[1] Part of the debate is on the question of whether physician-assisted suicide should be restricted to the former group or should also embrace the latter (see Martin Gunderson and David Mayo, "Restricting Physician-Assisted Death to the Terminally Ill," *Hastings Center Report* 30, no. 6 (2000): 17–23).

The observation that the debate on suicide assistance focuses on severely ill people has a legal side, too. The usual prototypes for the legalization of assisted suicide are in fact far off from providing a general legal right to receiving medical aid for committing suicide. Quite to the contrary, as a rule, physician-assisted suicide is illegal throughout the world.[2] There are only a few legal systems—for example, in Switzerland, Belgium, the Netherlands, and the US states of Oregon, Washington, Vermont, California, and Colorado—in which the complete prohibition is relaxed for a few very restricted cases and for an extremely small number of people.

The Washington Death with Dignity Act, issued by the State of Washington in 2008, states,

> An adult who is competent, is a resident of Washington state, and has been determined by the attending physician and consulting physician to be suffering from a terminal disease, and who has voluntarily expressed his or her wish to die, may make a written request for medication that the patient may self-administer to end his or her life in a humane and dignified manner in accordance with this chapter. (Chapter 70.245 RCW)

Thus, Washington state residents who are terminally ill can apply for a lethal drug in order to end their life. According to the Washington State Department of Health's 2010 annual report, 87 citizens participated in the program, 51 of whom died after ingesting the medication.[3] At the same time, however, in 2010 in Washington state, nearly 1,000 people committed suicide by other means, mostly by firearms, poison, and suffocation, and at least four times as many people attempted to kill themselves unsuccessfully.[4] Certainly, many of those people would have preferred the aid of medical professionals in killing themselves instead of doing it on their own. State law, however, would not allow them access to these facilities, not even in order to preserve their dignity.

---

[2] Strictly speaking, Germany is an exception because its penal law does not prohibit suicide assistance (except for special cases). However, professional regulations and legal duties for helping in emergency cases amount to a de facto prohibition of medical suicide assistance in non-medical instances.

[3] See http://www.doh.wa.gov/portals/1/Documents/Pubs/422-109-DeathWithDignityAct2015.pdf, accessed January 24, 2017.

[4] Washington State Department of Health, *Washington State Injury and Violence Prevention Guide*, 35–36, available online at www.doh.wa.gov/Portals/1/Documents/2900/InjuryReportFinal.pdf, accessed January 24, 2017.

The question is whether this legal restraint is ethically justifiable. If so, one could ask whether considerations that speak against a general right to physician-assisted suicide might also cast doubt on assisted suicide for severely ill patients.

Why should we distinguish between suicide assistance for very ill patients and that for other people who are weary of life? In a defense of the Oregon Death with Dignity Act, Ronald Lindsay, president of the secular Center for Inquiry, has addressed this question explicitly. "Respect for autonomy," he writes (I think that what he means is very close to respect for dignity), "is one reason for supporting legalization of assistance in dying, but it is not a sufficient reason."[5] He then lists some additional reasons in order to explain why only terminally ill patients should be provided with assistance in suicide. Here, I follow him partially and present some other reasons he does not mention.

His first reason is that it might not be necessary for other people. Typically, suicide is committed without any help. People shoot themselves, hang themselves, and poison themselves; they jump in front of trains or off of skyscrapers. So, why should anybody feel obliged to assist them? Terminally ill patients, on the other hand, are usually severely impaired in their possibilities to act. Most of them are confined to a bed or a wheelchair. Therefore, they need help to kill themselves.

This first reason for making the difference is not convincing, however. Although it is true that usually there are different alternatives for killing oneself, most of them are utterly immoral. They have awful side effects on other people—for example, on relatives who are the first to find the deceased, on the train conductor who helplessly watches his or her train hit the suicide attempter, or on passers-by who are suddenly confronted with a shattered corpse in front of a building. The fact that usually people are able to kill themselves without any medical help is therefore no justification for excluding them from assistance. To the contrary, such assistance could still be necessary for them to kill themselves in a morally acceptable way.

Second, one could be tempted to restrict physician-assisted suicide to terminally ill patients because as patients they obviously have to be cared for by physicians, whereas for other people, suicide is their own business. However, this is again a poor reason because, for example, soccer players are not patients either and yet physicians look after them as well. The same could be true for potential suicides.

---

[5] Ronald A. Lindsay, "Oregon's Experience: Evaluating the Record," *American Journal of Bioethics* 9, no. 3 (2009): 19–27, 20.

A third, much more interesting, reason for the differentiation follows from Lindsay's claim that the restriction of physician-assisted suicide to terminally ill patients can ensure that "a request for assistance in dying is not the product of some hasty, irrational decision."[6] This claim deserves careful consideration.

First, one might wonder whether the attitudes toward suicide held by patients at the very end of their lives are really not hasty but stable. Canadian psychiatrist Harvey Chochinov and colleagues investigated the temporal development of the will to live of cancer patients admitted to a palliative care program during an 18-month period in the mid-1990s. They concluded that the "will to live is highly unstable among terminally ill cancer patients."[7] Hence, according to the authors, "demonstration of the sustained wish to die must be part of evaluating any death-hastening request."[8] As with other suicidal persons, we should not take the patients' wish to end their lives as proof of a stable, reliable attitude. In this respect, there is no justification to distinguish between terminally ill patients and other people.

However, perhaps the crucial difference is not the stability but, rather, the rationality of the patients' decision to commit suicide. The idea that it might be irrational to end one's life is supported by one of the non-medical cases mentioned previously—the English nurse who killed herself because she felt so embarrassed by a prank. Although we understand why she ended her life, we hardly appreciate what she did. Merely being the victim of a silly joke is not so harmful for the dignity of one's further life that it would be appropriate to kill oneself. Hence, if someone had helped her—for example, provided her with the rope she used to commit suicide—we would not regard this assistance as legitimate. The nurse acted on a mistaken view of her dignity and its demands, and because we know better, it would have been wrong to support her misguided deed. A legal restriction of suicide assistance to severely ill patients would have prevented this wrongful help.

It is less clear, however, that the patients' wishes could not be equally misguided. At first glance, perhaps, one might assume that the patients' wish to die could not be as irrational as other people's wishes because these patients suffer so much that they certainly have an overwhelming

---

[6] Lindsay, "Oregon's Experience," 21.
[7] Harvey Max Chochinov, et al., "Will to Live in the Terminally Ill," *The Lancet* 354, no. 9181 (1999): 816–819, 818.
[8] Chochinov et al., "Will to Live in the Terminally Ill," 819.

reason to end their plight. There is empirical evidence against this presumption, however. Linda Ganzini and colleagues investigated the reasons why patients in Oregon request physician-assisted suicide.[9] Their study found that patients almost never request medical aid for suicide because of their actual state—of how they actually feel—but, rather, because of their expectations for their life in the future. They want to die because, for example, they do not want to become unable to control their situation, they do not want to suffer from terrible pain in the future, and—particularly important for my topic—they do not want to lose dignity. In another study, William Breitbart and colleagues confirmed these findings: "However, we found no significant association between desire for hastened death and either the presence of pain or pain intensity."[10] Hence, according to these data, it is not the patients' dreadful present that motivates them in asking for suicide aid, which probably would be a good reason beyond doubt; rather, it is the dreadful prospect they envisage.

Perhaps such a prospect could be as mistaken as the erroneous prospects of the London nurse, however. Palliative care and particularly what Harvey Chochinov called "dignity-conserving care" can uphold many of the elements of life that are particularly valuable for patients.[11] Given these opportunities, their decision to kill themselves may be as erroneous as the nurse's decision to hang herself. Therefore, if it is legitimate to protect non-terminally ill people from making such a fatal mistake, terminally ill patients deserve the same protection.

To be sure, matters are different in a situation in which the bleak expectations of the patients are not erroneous but realistic, because palliative treatment, although available in principle, is not accessible for the particular patients. Ronald Dworkin and colleagues express this possibility very clearly in their famous Philosopher's Brief from 1997, advocating the legalization of assisted suicide:

> The most important benefit of legalized assisted suicide for poor patients however, might be better care while they live. For though the medical experts cited in various briefs disagreed sharply about the percentage of terminal cases in which pain can be made tolerable through advanced and

[9] Linda Ganzini, Elizabeth R. Goy, and Steven K. Dobscha, "Oregonians' Reasons for Requesting Physician Aid in Dying," *Archives of Internal Medicine* 169, no. 5 (2009): 489–492.

[10] W. Breitbart, "Depression, Hopelessness, and Desire for Hastened Death in Terminally Ill Patients with Cancer," *JAMA* 284, no. 22 (2000): 2907–2911.

[11] Harvey Max Chochinov, "Dignity-Conserving Care—A New Model for Palliative Care: Helping the Patient Feel Valued," *JAMA* 287, no. 17 (2002): 2253–2260.

expensive palliative techniques, they did not disagree that a great many patients do not receive the relief they could have. The Solicitor General who urged the court to reverse the lower court judgments conceded in the oral argument that 25 percent of terminally ill patients actually do die in pain.[12]

If I understand the argument correctly, what the authors say is that because the poor cannot afford a proper treatment during their last days, giving them the opportunity to kill themselves early enough would allow them a painless death and, moreover, save a significant amount money that could be used for better treatment of the poor in general.

Prima facie, this is a strong conditional argument in favor of a legal option for assisted suicide for terminally ill patients. Given a society that cannot or does not afford a decent medical system, one might better allow for physician-assisted suicide than let many people die unaided. Physician-assisted suicide then would be a kind of voluntary, self-imposed mercy killing, and of course, there could be no serious argument against allowing it. Not allowing it would be like not giving von Tresckow the grenade and handing him over to Hitler's torturers instead.

Still, there is something very odd in the argumentation. This becomes evident when we compare it with another one of my previous examples. Unlike the London nurse, the raped Indian woman probably had a very realistic expectation about her future life. The author of a BBC report on the case concluded the following: "In the village, then, the notion that rape places a burden of shame on the shoulders of the survivor continues unchallenged. Geeta's death was, for many, inevitable." [13] Again, one could argue that because there is no realistic hope for a dignified life for raped women in India within the near future, at least the state should offer them a peaceful medical death in order to spare them the shameful existence they are envisioning. Moreover, the same might be considered, for example, for poor old people in Russia, handicapped children in Romania, or starving refugees from the civil wars of Africa. Because we will not help them live, we might at least help them die.

Evidently, what is wrong with these arguments is that they ignore the much stronger obligation to help these people live. Public measures such as the legalization of physician-assisted suicide are usually issued by the same institution that has the power to change the unbearable circumstances

---

[12] Ronald Dworkin et al., "Assisted Suicide: The Philosophers' Brief," *New York Review of Books*, March 27, 1997: 41–47.
[13] See http://www.bbc.com/news/magazine-37735370, accessed January 24, 2017.

under which some people live. Just like it is unacceptable for the Indian state to establish suicide assistance for raped women instead of fighting their discrimination, it is a moral scandal that presumably a large percentage of poor American citizens do not get the means for dying a decent death. What one needs in both cases is not support in committing suicide but, rather, a morally decent state doing its job.

So far, I have considered whether there may be reasons to restrain medical assistance in suicide only to a subgroup of people who want to end their lives in order to save their dignity, namely those who are severely ill. As it turns out, none of the reasons support such a differentiation. This leaves us with the presumption that everybody should have an option for suicide assistance.

However, as we have seen in the discussion of the third and fourth reasons, it is hardly advisable to provide such assistance unconditionally because sometimes people are wrong about the future challenge to their individual dignity, or even if they are correct, there may be other, morally superior ways for helping them.

It might be argued, however, that apart from such cases, there are still many situations in which people rightly assume that killing themselves would save them from leading undignified lives and in which there is no other way to help them other than to support their suicide. In order to examine this suggestion, it is advisable to take a closer look at the conception of dignity and its ethical relevance.

Dignity is a rather contested concept in moral philosophy. Although the previously discussed examples illustrate that from everyday moral life we are still familiar with the idea of doing something in order to protect our dignity and we certainly understand why dignity plays an important role for the Indian woman as well as for the London nurse, talking about dignity may still seem somewhat alien or old-fashioned. We occasionally use the term, but for most of us, it is not something we seem to care about much in everyday life. In a book review titled "The Stupidity of Dignity," American psychologist Stephen Pinker writes,

> In fact, every one of us voluntarily and repeatedly relinquishes dignity for other goods in life. Getting out of a small car is undignified. Having sex is undignified. Doffing your belt and spread-eagling to allow a security guard to slide a wand up your crotch is undignified. Most pointedly, modern medicine is a gantlet of indignities.[14]

---

[14] Steven Pinker, "The Stupidity of Dignity," *The New Republic* 238, May 28, 2008: 28–31.

Yet, if that were all there is to human dignity, then we had little reason to bother much about the relationship between assisted suicide and dignity. Therefore, the question is why we are so concerned about dignity in the ethics of assisted suicide at all.

In the literature, it is quite common to answer this question by distinguishing two different concepts of dignity.[15] The first is human dignity, which is mentioned in in the preamble of the *Charter of the United Nations*, in the *Universal Declaration of Human Rights*, and also in the first article of the German *Grundgesetz*. Human dignity represents our fundamental moral status, our basic claim to being respected in our human rights—particularly our right to life. The second is contingent dignity, which is a matter of inherited or acquired status and social approval. One's contingent dignity usually is dependent on one's own behavior and on how one is treated by others. Whereas human dignity is inviolable, inalienable, and of utmost importance for ethics, contingent dignity is what one may risk in having sex, getting out of small cars, or passing the security controls at the airport (as Pinker reminded us) and is comparably less important.

This distinction between two concepts of dignity is much too simple, however, historically as well as systematically. It is true that a hit to one's contingent social dignity may sometimes be tolerable and unimportant. Yet, not losing one's contingent dignity as a whole is of utmost importance for all of us. Survivors of concentration camps, torture, and rape occasionally report how devastating humiliation and degradation can be and that these may feel worst of all plights.[16] It was under the impression of these experiences that the concept of human dignity entered the legal scene after World War II. The duty to respect someone's human dignity, therefore, is much more specific than the bold claim that one should obey his or her fundamental rights. It is the duty not to strip a person of her social identity, her contingent dignity.[17] The duty is relatively moderate with respect to

---

[15] For a sophisticated version of this claim, see Michael Rosen, *Dignity: Its History and Meaning* (Cambridge, Mass.: Harvard University Press, 2012).

[16] Terrence Des Pres, *The Survivor: An Anatomy of Life in the Death Camps* (New York: Oxford University Press, 1976).

[17] For an elaboration of this conception of human dignity, see Ralf Stoecker, "Three Crucial Turns on the Road to an Adequate Understanding of Human Dignity," in *Violations of Human Dignity*, ed. by Paulus Kaufmann et al. (Dordrecht: Springer, 2010), 7–19; Christian Neuhäuser and Ralf Stoecker, "Human Dignity as Universal Nobility," in *The Cambridge Handbook of Human Dignity: Inter-disciplinary Perspectives*, ed. by Marcus Duwell et al. (Cambridge: Cambridge University Press, 2014), 298–309. A similar view has been proposed by Jeremy Waldron (Jeremy Waldron, *Dignity, Rank, and Rights* (New York: Oxford University Press, 2012)).

minor offenses, but it becomes overriding when challenging the victim's whole identity.

Human dignity, according to this proposal, is not a special kind of dignity; rather, it stands for the general value of having one's contingent dignity respected and supported. Because human dignity is not a dignity in itself, it obviously cannot be diminished or forfeited. In this sense, it is inborn and inviolable. Still, it can be respected or disdained depending on the way a person's contingent dignity is respected or violated.

Such an understanding of human dignity is not only historically plausible but also has the advantage of meeting the objection that dignity is an old-fashioned concept. Although the term "dignity" might be outdated, the basic conception is not. A large variety of words and expressions that express similar ideas are still in frequent use, from "saving one's countenance" or "feeling embarrassed" to being "hip" or "uncool." We still know very well how these normative concepts work and how they are related to respect and disdain, pride and shame, humiliation and degradation.

What has changed since the time of the Trojan War, however, are the contents of dignity: They have become much more variable and group specific. We allow for numerous ways of creating an individual identity. Yet, it is still us, the social group, who define the boundaries of dignity. Dignity is still subject to social determination. As individuals, we are not free in deciding what dignity demands. It is as members of the society that we argue about what is dignified and what is not. Moreover, we argue about ways of protecting and restoring dignity in special circumstances—for example, about how to deal with grave humiliations and what we expect from people whose dignities have been harmed. No doubt, there is much disagreement about these questions, and people take their pride and dignity in matters that others disregard as worthless. What is important for the topic under consideration, however, is that we are not willing simply to accept whatever it is that someone takes to be dignified as a cause for supporting him or her. Respecting a person's human dignity does not compel us to share his or her view on where dignity lies. Instead, we might claim that this person is wrong about his or her dignity.

This is what we would say about the British nurse. Although she was embarrassed by the bad joke, it was neither necessary nor appropriate for retaining her dignity that she kill herself. In this respect, our views on the demands of dignity have changed considerably since the times of Ajax and Lucretia. In fact, in our society we usually assume that, to return to Seneca, we do not need exits from life anymore to preserve our dignity. To quote the famous Town Musicians of Bremen in one of the Grimm's fairy tales: "Something better than death we can find anywhere." Although we understand that things have been different in antiquity and that dire circumstances such as being a resistance fighter under the Nazi regime can change things, too, we are convinced that in our society dignity never should make it reasonable for someone to kill herself or himself, whether the person has been raped, is a scorned lover, is bankrupt, or is suffering from bullying. Hence, considerations of dignity do not compel us into legalization of physician-assisted suicide for any of these persons. This is why we would not have helped the British nurse kill herself in order to wipe out the shame inflicted to her by the prank.

If I am right with this observation about our widely shared conception of what dignity demands, we face the crucial question whether this should be different for people at the ends of their lives. Should we make a fundamental distinction between the Town Musicians' attitudes regarding our ordinary view on living in dignity, according to which there is always another dignified alternative to death, and a special exception for people under certain medical conditions? I believe there are at least two good reasons to answer this question in the negative.

The first reason against the distinction is that one cannot accept that someone preserves his or her dignity by committing suicide without indicating a judgment upon other people in a similar situation who act otherwise. This is the background for why we would regard it as absurd if the Indian government would establish assisted suicide as an option for mistreated women in order to help them save their dignity. It would amount to the concession that other mistreated women who stay alive live in degradation. In antiquity, this was the lesson to be learned from Lucretia: There is no decent life for women after rape. But this lesson is evidently incorrect. It is not the innocent victim who should be forced to live on in shame but, rather, the culprit. Not only individuals, such as the British nurse, but also whole societies, such as the ancient Greek or modern Indian societies, can have mistaken conceptions of dignity and shame. Because these are mistaken views, however, they cannot justify institutional support for citizens who have difficulty meeting the demands of the outdated codex.

If we transfer these considerations to the situation of patients at the ends of their lives, we have to conclude that justifying the legalization of assisted suicide on the grounds of dignity is by necessity degrading for those patients who do not want to kill themselves, too. As soon as suicide is regarded as a necessary means for maintaining one's dignity, then forgoing it is shameful. Hence, advocates of a legal right to assisted suicide confront a dilemma: Either they accept that patients really can be right to regard the continuation of their lives as undignified, and thus they must maintain that other patients in similar situations who do not kill themselves behave undignified, or they abstain from any judgment about the correctness of the patients' views about their dignity, in which case they need an argument as to why suicide assistance still should be provided. It seems to me that both horns of the dilemma are rather uncomfortable.

Moreover, there is a second reason that speaks against the idea that we should accept that in the case of terminal illness, unlike all other situations in life, dignity might demand killing oneself. It is connected to the very first argument presented in this chapter, according to which withholding a person necessary aid for killing herself violates her dignity because it interferes with her right to self-determination. This is a very strong argument because the right to self-determination certainly is a core element of dignity. Restrictions on the way we live always endanger our pride, particularly when they touch upon existential questions such as how we are going to die. These are paradigmatically private questions. They concern our self-understanding and self-respect. How could someone, even the state, dare to interfere? As stated previously, this is a very strong reason against any legal prohibition of medical suicide assistance. It is a demand of autonomy as part of our dignity not to inhibit our opportunity to end our lives at will.

However, there is another, more skeptical consideration connected to this argument, which leads back to the relationship between suicide assistance and the dignity of those who might not want to kill themselves. Usually, it is assumed that opening up choices for someone is increasing her autonomy and thereby strengthening her dignity. Yet, this is not always true; an offer for choice can also be humiliating in itself. The paradigmatic example is Sophie's Choice, a situation taken from the book by William Styron in which a sadistic Nazi asks a mother to choose which of her two children he should condemn to death. By opening up this choice, he is not in any way doing Sophie a favor—nor is it meant so. Instead, it is a particularly cruel way of torturing her because it burdens her with the load of responsibility for whatever it is she chooses. Whether she decides for one or the other child, in any case she has to live with the knowledge that sending one of her children to death was not merely something inflicted on her but also something she did. And there is hardly anything conceivable that could be a heavier burden on someone's identity and hence be more humiliating than this.

Of course, terminally ill patients are not in the situation of a desperate mother in a concentration camp. However, as soon as we open up a legal opportunity for these patients to get medical aid for committing suicide, then inevitably they become responsible, too, for either grasping the opportunity or continuing to live. Occasionally, these patients are a burden for their relatives, and they know that they are a burden and are very concerned about it. Christine McPherson and colleagues, who have explored the perspectives of patients at the end of life, summarize their results as follows: "Self-perceived burden has emerged as a major concern for many people who are nearing the end of life."[18] Given the possibility of assisted suicide, however, the suffering of the relatives is not just bad luck anymore but also inflicted on them by the patients who do not choose to end their lives in a timely manner.

That these patients feel responsible for their family's plight is already a wretched situation for them, and in this respect it is an obstacle for a decent death. However, their responsibility also has a moral aspect. It might very well be that a detached calculation of the advantages and disadvantages of their choice will lead to the conclusion that the negative consequences for the relatives are so severe and that the remaining quality of the patients' lives is so poor in comparison that they find themselves obliged to commit suicide. And they might even be right. As soon as society establishes an opportunity to choose medical aid in killing themselves, patients are confronted with the moral question of whether they have a duty to accept the offer. In the public debate, this possibility usually plays no role at all; it is always assumed that a choice for ending one's life could be based on purely egoistic grounds. However, egoism is not a plausible ethical theory, and in all other normative systems, one's fellow people also have to enter into one's deliberation. It is not clear, however, that one may then be able to justify continuing to live.

As stated previously, I assume that it is part of our understanding of dignity that for everybody—no matter what he or she has done or whatever he or she has suffered—there is a decent way to go on living and no necessity to end one's life. From this perspective, however, it would be deeply embarrassing for severely ill people if they were compelled to justify why they do not kill themselves and perhaps were not even able to provide such a justification. This is the second reason why we should not regard the

[18] Christine J. McPherson, Keith G. Wilson, and Mary Ann Murray, "Feeling Like a Burden: Exploring the Perspectives of Patients at the End of Life," *Social Science & Medicine* 64, no. 2 (2007): 417–427, 424. There are probably cultural variations, though. See Tatsuya Morita et al., "Desire for Death and Requests to Hasten Death of Japanese Terminally Ill Cancer Patients Receiving Specialized Inpatient Palliative Care," *Journal of Pain and Symptom Management* 27, no. 1 (2004): 44–52, 49.

legalization of assisted suicide as a means to promote a more dignified life for ill patients. Such a measure might threaten the dignity of those patients who would not like to shorten their lives.

Now we seem to be stuck, however, between considerations that speak against the idea of suicide as one possible way of dying with dignity and worries that the establishment of assisted suicide might violate third parties' dignity, on the one hand, and the claim that dignity demands respecting the right to self-determination, part of which is the liberty to kill oneself, on the other hand.

Fortunately, these views are not really in conflict. Instead, they point to a situation that is quite familiar to us. Even if someone has a distorted view about what it means to live a decent life, we usually feel obliged to respect his or her autonomy and hence do not interfere. A young man who decides to spend his life worshipping an Indian guru presumably is wrong. However, it would be offending his dignity to detain him from traveling to India. What we could and should do instead is to argue with him in order to persuade him to change his mind and make very clear that we regard his decision as erroneous. Moreover, we would not feel too much obliged to assist him in his plans.

To my mind, this is just what is necessary with respect to medical suicide assistance. One has to maintain that suicide should not be regarded as part of dying with dignity. Unlike in other times and under different circumstances, we never should feel the need to end our lives in order to keep or restore our dignity. To the contrary, this assumption is deeply humiliating for other people in the same situation. Therefore, people should not choose suicide assistance on the grounds of dignity. They are wrong if they do so. However, inhibiting their choice, even if they are wrong, would violate their right to self-determination and hence be humiliating. It would not impair their dying with dignity but, rather, their living with dignity. Consequently, there should not be a legal prohibition of medical assistance for suicide. Further measures, however—for example, the institutionalization of suicide assistance—should be checked for their potential to put pressure on all ill patients by compelling them to either accept suicide assistance or actively decide for a continuation of their lives (including all negative side effects).

In a sense, this argument is orthogonal to the received positions in the debate. There are those who defend assisted suicide as a means for dying with dignity and therefore plead for its legalization. Others respect it as a possible way of ending one's life but have difficulties with the legal allowance of medical support. Finally, there are those who reject it as part of dying with dignity and infer that it should be legally prohibited. According to my view, the person herself should not end her life voluntarily. In particular, she should not regard suicide as a demand of dignity. Thus, I am in agreement with the defenders of the third position (although on somewhat different grounds). However, because it is the agent's very personal matter whether she kills herself, we can at best try to persuade her but must not interfere. In this regard, I am with the former positions. From an ethical perspective, society should not legally prohibit physician-assisted suicide, but at the same time, society should ensure that suicide is neither necessary nor appropriate for leading a decent life up to its very end.

SECTION 2 | Dignity at the End of Life

CHAPTER 4 | Dignity through Thick and Thin

L. W. SUMNER

I AM PERHAPS not ideally qualified to discuss the role of human dignity in assisted death. After all, I managed to write a fairly lengthy and (as I thought) pretty thorough treatment of the ethical and legal status of physician-assisted death with scarcely a mention of dignity.[1] The two values I invoked in the course of defending the ethics of assisted death were patient well-being and patient autonomy. In making this case, I saw no need to give separate attention to dignity. The one entry for "dignity" in my index refers readers to my critique of some arguments by David Velleman, who relies on a conception of human dignity in building a case against the permissibility of suicide (and, perforce, assisted suicide and euthanasia). Velleman obviously thought that his arguments could not go through without this appeal to dignity; equally obviously, I thought mine could.

I have since come to think that I should have given dignity a little more airtime for the role it might play on my side of the debate. So one of my purposes here is to advance a kind of corrective to the arguments of the book, one that is somewhat more accommodating of dignity. It will not alter the central features of those arguments, and it certainly will not alter their conclusions, but it might make those arguments and conclusions a little more appealing to those with a better feel for the importance of dignity than I had.

In attempting to recuperate dignity for my cause, I am at odds with those critics who have argued that the concept has outlived whatever usefulness

---

[1] L. W. Sumner, *Assisted Death: A Study in Ethics and Law* (New York: Oxford University Press, 2011).

it ever had, at least in bioethics. Ruth Macklin has famously contended that dignity is a "useless concept."[2] Appeals to dignity, she contends, are either empty or redundant. They are empty—"mere slogans"—if, as is so often the case, dignity remains undefined. The leading examples of this neglect are those international instruments—declarations, covenants, conventions, and so on—in which dignity is invoked as the foundation of human rights. Article 1 of the *Universal Declaration of Human Rights* (1948) begins with the sentence, "All human beings are born free and equal in dignity and rights," and the *International Covenant on Economic, Social and Cultural Rights* and the *International Covenant on Civil and Political Rights* (1966) both state that all human rights derive from the inherent dignity of the human person.[3] Needless to say, these instruments, and many others like them, do not pause to add any flesh to the bare bones of dignity. Nor are similar documents with specific application to bioethics any more forthcoming. The Council of Europe's *Convention on Human Rights and Biomedicine* (1997) states as its fundamental principle that "parties to this Convention shall protect the dignity and identity of all human beings,"[4] and one of the stated aims of the UNESCO *Universal Declaration on Bioethics and Human Rights* (2005) is "to promote respect for human dignity and protect human rights."[5]

The complete absence of any elaboration or definition of the concept in these instruments has led some commentators to conclude that it has mere placeholder status: "Dignity" is the convenient label for the unknown X—whatever it is—that is the basis for possession of universal human rights.[6] Giving the concept more determinate content, moreover, would be counterproductive because it would reduce the likelihood of achieving overlapping consensus on a list of specific rights. It is far easier to secure agreement, for instance, on a clause prohibiting torture than on

---

[2] Ruth Macklin, "Dignity Is a Useless Concept," *British Medical Journal* 327, no. 7429 (2003): 1419–1420. For a more recent assault on the concept, as it is sometimes deployed in bioethical contexts, see Steven Pinker, "The Stupidity of Dignity," *The New Republic* 238 (May 28, 2008): 28–31.

[3] For these and many more such instruments, see Christopher McCrudden, "Human Dignity and Judicial Interpretation of Human Rights," *European Journal of International Law* 19, no. 4 (2008): 655–724.

[4] http://www.coe.int/en/web/conventions/full-list/-/conventions/rms/090000168007cf98, accessed December 14, 2016.

[5] http://portal.unesco.org/en/ev.php-URL_ID=31058&URL_DO=DO_TOPIC&URL_SECTION=201.html, accessed December 14, 2016.

[6] McCrudden, "Human Dignity and Judicial Interpretation of Human Rights," 675–678; David Luban, "Human Dignity, Humiliation, and Torture," *Kennedy Institute of Ethics Journal* 19, no. 3 (2009): 211–230.

any particular theory explaining what, exactly, is wrong with the practice. "Dignity," as Jeremy Waldron has observed, is a "feel-good word"; everyone is in favor of respecting human dignity, although they may have very different conceptions of what it is.[7] It shares this positive but malleable connotation with other feel-good words, such as "freedom," "democracy," and "justice." Leaving dignity "undertheorized" in human rights instruments therefore allows all parties to the agreement to assume their own favored understanding of what it means while converging on a common list of practices that it either requires or prohibits.

So much grist for Macklin's mill: In these contexts, dignity does seem little more than an empty slogan. Sometimes, however, it is given some genuine content. The Canadian *Tri-Council Policy Statement: Ethical Conduct for Research Involving Humans* (2014) begins with the familiar declaration: "Respect for human dignity requires that research involving humans be conducted in a manner that is sensitive to the inherent worth of all human beings and the respect and consideration that they are due." However, it immediately concedes that "the term lends itself to a variety of definitions and interpretations that make it challenging to apply" and goes on to specify that "respect for human dignity is expressed through three core principles—respect for persons, concern for welfare, and justice." The three principles are familiar in bioethics: Respect for persons requires the protection of individual autonomy, concern for welfare means pretty much what it says, and justice involves treating research subjects fairly and equitably. The statement then provides an extensive explication of each of these principles, eventually devoting approximately 200 pages to spelling out the obligations that researchers owe to their subjects, all in the name of dignity.[8]

The concept of dignity, therefore, need not be empty. But by giving it content, the statement exposes itself to Macklin's other charge of redundancy. Dignity, she claims, turns out to mean nothing more than respect for persons or for their autonomy. To be fair, the Tri-Council statement gives it a little wider scope because it also includes safeguarding the well-being of research subjects and treating them fairly. But Macklin's main complaint stands: Once we bring these principles into play, we do not need the concept of dignity except as a convenient umbrella term or as

---

[7] Jeremy Waldron, *The Harm in Hate Speech* (Cambridge, Mass.: Harvard University Press, 2012), 137.
[8] http://www.pre.ethics.gc.ca/pdf/eng/tcps2-2014/TCPS_2_FINAL_Web.pdf, accessed December 14, 2016.

honorific window dressing. Instead of blathering on about dignity, let's just go directly to autonomy, well-being, and fairness.

If we are not to side with Macklin and give up taking dignity seriously, the challenge is clear: to find a working conception of the abstract concept that (1) has some distinctive content of its own and (2) has some real work to do in bioethics—specifically, in debates about assisted death. Dignity, of course, has an annoying habit of turning up on both sides of those debates. I have already noted Velleman's use of it to condemn suicide. Within the "right to die" community, however, "death with dignity" is the common euphemism for physician-assisted dying. Given the status of dignity as a feel-good concept, this adaptability is not surprising. Nor is it necessarily a strike against it: It is entirely possible that physician-assisted death might both compromise and enhance dignity, especially if, as seems likely, "dignity" is used in different senses by the parties on either side. But it does encourage the suspicion that, as Waldron states, dignity is "a mushy word" that "might mean anything."[9]

The standard response to Macklin's challenge is to distinguish different senses of "dignity" and to argue that some of these senses, at least, are both distinctive and useful in bioethical debates.[10] Philosophers love to draw distinctions, and I am not immune to the charms of this pastime. However, I am going to proceed in a slightly different way. I will make no attempt to catalog all of the possible conceptions of the concept, focusing instead on those that are particularly germane to the end-of-life debates. Here, I think that it is useful to array these conceptions on a scale from thin to thick. Following the usual convention, I consider that a concept's degree of thickness is a function of the amount of empirical content that it marries to its evaluative content. At the one extreme, a concept is thin if it is purely evaluative with little or no empirical content. The standard examples are "good" and "bad" and "right" and "wrong," which do not include the empirical grounds of their application. At the other extreme, it is thick if it is rich in such content. Familiar virtues and vices such as

---

[9] Waldron, *The Harm in Hate Speech*, 139. Waldron also notes that "dignity discourse is cursed by equivocation." This does not prevent him from invoking a conception of dignity in his defense of hate speech laws. Nor should it.

[10] Doris Schroeder, "Dignity: Two Riddles and Four Concepts," *Cambridge Quarterly of Healthcare Ethics* 17, no. 2 (2008): 230–238; Rieke van der Graaf and Johannes J. M. van Delden, "Clarifying Appeals to Dignity in Medical Ethics from an Historical Perspective," *Bioethics* 23, no. 3 (2009): 151–160; Suzy Killmister, "Dignity: Not Such a Useless Concept," *Journal of Medical Ethics* 36, no. 3 (2010): 160–164; Stephen W. Smith, *End-of-Life Decisions in Medical Care: Principles and Policies for Regulating the Dying Process* (Cambridge: Cambridge University Press, 2012), chap. 7.

honesty and dishonesty, generosity, and meanness tend toward this end of the scale. And, of course, there are intermediate possibilities. I argue that conceptions of dignity can also be either thick or thin and that in considering the ethics of assisted death we have reason to prefer the thick to the thin.[11]

In the various human rights documents cited previously, we already have on board some examples of a conception of dignity that tends toward the thin end. In those documents, dignity seems to be the placeholder for whatever it is about humans (or persons) in virtue of which they have rights. As such, it presumably gestures toward some special value, or importance, or status that humans (or persons) have. Even this conception is not entirely devoid of empirical content because although we are not told what it is about humans (or persons) in virtue of which they have this special value, at least we know that it is not shared with non-humans (or non-persons). But there seems to be little added, beyond rhetorical effect, by labeling this value "dignity." This becomes clear when, in discussions of the basis of human rights, "dignity" comes to be used interchangeably with "worth."[12] If human dignity is just a special kind of value or worth that humans (or persons) have, then why not just stick with the (thin) value concept?

This thin notion of dignity is frequently labeled Kantian, which takes us back again to David Velleman, who invokes it in his argument against suicide. Velleman's strategy turns on a distinction between two different kinds of value pertaining to persons.[13] The first is the value of a person's life *for that person*, which is identical to her well-being. It is this value we have in mind when we talk about someone's interest or good or say that her life is going well or badly for her. The second kind of value belongs to all persons by virtue of some property or capacity inherent in their nature;

---

[11] Margaret Battin draws a similar distinction between conceptions of dignity, which she labels as Kantian and empirical: Margaret Pabst Battin, *The Least Worst Death: Essays in Bioethics on the End of Life* (New York: Oxford University Press, 1994), 282. However, these labels suggest that "empirical dignity" is not an evaluative concept. For that reason, I prefer to treat it as a thick evaluative concept rich in empirical content.

[12] William T. Blackstone, "Human Rights and Human Dignity," *Philosophical Forum* 9, no. 1–2 (1971): 3–37, 34–35: Human rights are based on "the principle that humans are beings with intrinsic worth and dignity." Herbert Spiegelberg, "Human Dignity: A Challenge to Contemporary Philosophy," *Philosophical Forum* 9, no. 1–2 (1971): 39–64, 59: "Human dignity is the worth of a person who is worth being for his own sake, regardless of his usefulness for another. It is because of this worth that he is worthy of personal respect."

[13] J. David Velleman, "A Right of Self-Termination?", *Ethics* 109, no. 3 (1999): 606–628. Cf. Jeff McMahan, *The Ethics of Killing: Problems at the Margins of Life* (New York: Oxford University Press, 2002), 241.

this is the notion that, following Kant, Velleman calls dignity, and it is for him the secular version of the sanctity of human life. What morality requires, Velleman claims, is that we respect the dignity of persons, which includes respecting our own dignity. Suicide, whether physician-assisted or otherwise, may well be in the best interest of a patient suffering through the end stages of an incurable illness. But deciding for suicide just on this basis would be impermissible, Velleman argues, because it would disrespect the patient's dignity as a person.[14]

Velleman's argument that persons have this second kind of value runs as follows: "What's good for a person is worth caring about only out of concern for the person, and hence only insofar as he is worth caring about. A person's good has only hypothetical or conditional value, which depends on the value of the person himself."[15] So the case for dignity as a distinct value inhering in a person is that it is presupposed, and thus entailed, by the value of that person's interest. The same relation of dependence explains why it is not commensurable with, and therefore cannot be traded off against, the value of relief of suffering. Because dignity is the ground of the value of well-being, it has lexical priority over it. Suicide for the purpose of preventing further suffering, whether assisted or otherwise, is therefore always wrong.

I have criticized this argument of Velleman's elsewhere and will not repeat that criticism here.[16] My present point is a much more modest one, namely that the concept of dignity plays no substantive role in the argument. "Dignity" for Velleman is just a label, an honorific, designed to make the kind of value he is invoking look particularly weighty or important. The substantive issue is whether or not persons have this kind of value and whether or not Velleman's argument shows that they do (I think not). Labeling the value "dignity" adds nothing to the argument. This is equally clear in the Kantian source from which Velleman is borrowing:

---

[14] Velleman allows that there may be other grounds for suicide compatible with respect for personal dignity; his objection is to suicide chosen solely on the ground that death would be best for the person in question. Presumably this objection would hold equally strongly for the decision to refuse life-sustaining treatment on the same ground. Velleman also allows that suffering can rise to the level at which it can justify suicide, but only if (and because) it undermines the capacity for rational agency (Velleman, "A Right of Self-Termination?", 618). This is a particularly perverse result because it means that by the time a patient's suffering has reached the point at which an assisted suicide would be justified, she has also lost the capacity for rational agency and so cannot autonomously request it. Some might regard this as a *reductio* of the view.

[15] Velleman, "A Right of Self-Termination?", 611. See 615: "We cannot avoid presupposing the existence of this value . . . since its needed to account for the importance of interest-relative values."

[16] Sumner, *Assisted Death*, 82–84.

In the kingdom of ends everything has either value or dignity. Whatever has a value can be replaced by something else which is equivalent; whatever, on the other hand, is above all value, and therefore admits of no equivalent, has a dignity. Whatever has reference to the general inclinations and wants of mankind has a market value; . . . but that which constitutes the condition under which alone anything can be an end in itself, this has not merely a relative worth, i.e., value, but an intrinsic worth, that is, dignity. Now morality is the condition under which alone a rational being can be an end in himself, since by this alone is it possible that he should be a legislating member in the kingdom of ends. Thus morality, and humanity as capable of it, is that which alone has dignity.[17]

The contrast that Kant is here drawing is between *Wert* ("value," sometimes rendered as "price"), which is fungible, and *Würde* ("dignity," sometimes rendered as "worth"), which is not. Dignity, for Kant, means nothing more than this special kind of value he thinks inheres in rational beings as legislators of the moral law, a value that establishes them as ends in themselves.

This Kantian conception of dignity (or worth) is thin, but it is not empty. Far from it: In the form explicated by Kant and Velleman, it is chock-full of normative content, robust enough to have lexical priority over competing kinds of value and to license a very strong, virtually exceptionless, prohibition of suicide and physician-assisted death. It is therefore not susceptible to Macklin's complaint about emptiness. But it is susceptible to her other complaint about redundancy. There is nothing in the conception of Kantian dignity that cannot be captured equally well just using the language of value or worth. As the first meaning of "dignity," the *Oxford English Dictionary* (*OED*) gives "the quality of being worthy or honourable; worthiness, worth, nobleness, excellence." So it is not arbitrary to use the language of dignity to mark the special status that Kant and Velleman want to attribute to rational beings, but it is not informative either.

Thus far, we have examined the conception of dignity invoked by what we may call the anti-choice side of the debate over assisted death—those who deny that patients have a moral right to this option. It is now time to examine more closely the pro-choice side. Here, dignity talk is ubiquitous, in enabling legislation (the Death with Dignity Acts in Oregon and Washington), in advocacy groups (e.g., the Canadian group Dying with

---

[17] Immanuel Kant, *Groundwork of the Metaphysics of Morals*, ed. Mary Gregor and Jens Timmerman (Cambridge: Cambridge University Press, 1998), 42–43.

Dignity), and most prominently in the Swiss assisted suicide organization Dignitas. This side also has a thin conception of dignity, in which a death with dignity is just synonymous with a good death. Everyone agrees that a good death (or, more accurately, a good dying) is a good thing—something to be aimed at in the case of individual patients and a worthy goal of end-of-life care. The notion of a good death is plainly thin because it gives us no information concerning the good-making properties of a death (or a dying). When "death with dignity" is simply used as a convenient sound bite, it too is thin—indeed, not just thin but (in Macklin's terms) empty. Dignity is not one particular good-making property of a death (very likely among others); instead, it is just another way of saying that the dying process went well, or at least as well as could be hoped.

We can, however, do rather better on this side of the question: We can listen to patients who say that they want a dignified death (or that they want to avoid at least some of the common indignities of the dying process). From available data, we know that the preservation of dignity is one of the main concerns of patients who elect an assisted death. The Oregon Public Health Division publishes annual statistical reports on the operation of the Death with Dignity Act.[18] These reports break down the number of patients who have utilized the provisions of the Act in the previous calendar year along several dimensions, such as sex, age, race, underlying illness, and so on. It also lists these patients' end-of-life concerns—the ones that motivated them to seek an assisted suicide. In rank order from most to least frequently cited, they are loss of autonomy, diminishing ability to engage in the activities that make life enjoyable, loss of dignity, loss of control of bodily functions, being a burden on family or caregivers, inadequate pain control, and the financial implications of treatment. Loss of dignity here ranks high, being cited in the case of more than 80% of patients. It seems clear from these reports that as far as patients are concerned, loss of dignity is one significant factor, although not the only one, that they seek to avoid in the dying process.[19] Turning this toward the positive, they seem to be voicing the view that the preservation of dignity is an important part of a good death.

However, considered as evidence of patient end-of-life concerns, the Oregon annual reports have some significant drawbacks. Principal

---

[18] https://public.health.oregon.gov/ProviderPartnerResources/EvaluationResearch/
DeathwithDignityAct/Pages/ar-index.aspx, accessed December 14, 2016.
[19] Comparable results have been reported by the Washington State Department of Health under the terms of the Washington Death with Dignity Act. http://www.doh.wa.gov/YouandYourFamily/IllnessandDisease/DeathwithDignityAct/DeathwithDignityData, accessed December 14, 2016.

among them is the fact that those concerns are not voiced directly by the patients themselves. The Oregon law requires patients to submit a written "Request for Medication to End My Life in a Human and Dignified Manner." However, it does not require them to provide any reason for this request. For any patient who dies as a result of ingesting the medication, the attending physician must submit a follow-up report that records, inter alia, the concerns that motivated the request for the prescription. For this, the physician is given a checklist of the seven aforementioned concerns, each of which requires a response of "Yes," "No," or "Don't Know." What we have in the annual reports, therefore, is an aggregate of the motivating reasons that doctors attribute to their patients, on the basis of whatever direct information they might have, these reasons being selected from a predetermined list.[20]

Fortunately, we also have more reliable evidence. Since its inception in 1997, the operation of the Oregon Death with Dignity Act has been extensively studied by Dr. Linda Ganzini and colleagues. In 2008, Ganzini et al. published the results of a survey in which they asked family members of decedents who had requested a physician-assisted death to rank twenty-eight possible reasons their loved ones made the request.[21] Ganzini et al.'s apparent assumption was that family members might have more intimate knowledge of the patient's motives and values than did the attending health care professionals. Of the twenty-eight possible reasons, loss of dignity ranked fourth.[22] In a study published in 2009, Ganzini et al. then applied the same methodology to persons who had either requested a physician-assisted death or contacted an advocacy organization (Compassion and

[20] Data for the Netherlands, also derived from doctors' reports, can be found in Marijke C. Jansen-van der Weide, Bregje D. Onwuteaka-Philipsen, and Gerrit van der Wal, "Granted, Undecided, Withdrawn, and Refused Requests for Euthanasia and Physician-Assisted Suicide," *Archives of Internal Medicine* 165, no. 15 (2005): 1698–1704; John Griffiths, Heleen Weyers, and Maurice Adams, *Euthanasia and Law in Europe* (Portland, Ore.: Hart Publishing, 2008), 169–170; Jojanneke E. van Alphen, Ge A. Donker, and Richard L. Marquet, "Requests for Euthanasia in General Practice before and after Implementation of the Dutch Euthanasia Act," *British Journal of General Practice* 60, no. 573 (2010): 263–267. There, too, loss of dignity ranks high among reported patient reasons for choosing an assisted death.

[21] Linda Ganzini, Elizabeth R. Goy, and Steven K. Dobscha, "Why Oregon Patients Request Assisted Death: Family Members' Views," *Journal of General Internal Medicine* 23, no. 2 (2008): 154–157.

[22] In a similar survey of family members of patients who had requested a physician-assisted death in the Netherlands, loss of dignity was cited as the most important reason for the request; Jean-Jacques Georges et al., "Relatives' Perspective on the Terminally Ill Patients Who Died after Euthanasia or Physician-Assisted Suicide: A Retrospective Cross-Sectional Interview Study in the Netherlands," *Death Studies* 31, no. 1 (2007): 1–15.

Choices of Oregon) for information about the process.[23] This time, loss of dignity ranked ninth on the list. It seems safe to conclude, therefore, that one important consideration motivating patients to seek a physician-assisted death is the wish to maintain their dignity or the fear that they might otherwise lose it.

This result, however, does not tell us what these patients considered dignity to be or what they thought might threaten it. These further questions were explored in an important study conducted by Dr. Harvey Chochinov and colleagues in which a cohort of patients terminally ill with cancer were asked to rate their sense of dignity.[24] Within that cohort, a relatively small minority indicated that they were experiencing an impaired sense of dignity. Factors contributing to this experience included (1) loss of autonomy or independence, largely resulting from confinement in a health care institution; (2) deterioration in personal appearance; (3) the need for assistance with intimate functions such as bathing and toileting; and (4) experiencing uncontrolled pain.

This empirical result points us toward two important lessons about the role of dignity at the end of life. The first is that it is not a stand-alone concern for patients. Recall the Oregon list of possible reasons for patients to request a physician-assisted death—loss of autonomy, loss of dignity, loss of control of bodily functions, inadequate pain control, and so on. For any given patient who has died as a result of such a request, more than one of these concerns may be listed as a motivating factor. What the Chochinov study shows is that some of the other items on the list may matter for a patient not only in their own right but also because they contribute to loss of dignity. Believing that one has no control over the direction of the dying process—that it is being driven by the course of the illness or by decisions made by others—may itself be experienced as an indignity. So might dependence on others for the simplest bodily functions—the kind of dependence associated with infancy—or being overwhelmed by pain or by other intractable physical symptoms such as nausea or shortness of breath. If this interdependence between dignity and some of the other factors is real, as the Chochinov study seems to show, then even the high ranking of loss of dignity as a motivating factor for patients who seek medical aid in dying may understate its importance. It is possible that most, even all, of

[23] Linda Ganzini, Elizabeth R. Goy, and Steven K. Dobscha, "Oregonians' Reasons for Requesting Physician Aid in Dying," *Archives of Internal Medicine* 169, no. 5 (2009): 489–492.
[24] Harvey Max Chochinov et al., "Dignity in the Terminally Ill: A Cross-Sectional, Cohort Study," *The Lancet* 360, no. 9350 (2002): 2026–2030.

the concerns that patients voice at the end of life matter to them at least in part because they are experienced as compromising their dignity.

The second lesson is that we can now begin to piece together what patients in end-of-life care mean by dignity. The Chochinov study reported that patients associated an impaired sense of dignity with "a feeling of being degraded, ashamed, or embarrassed." It went on to assert that each of the factors contributing to this impairment of dignity

> is associated with an altered sense of personal competence and autonomy and, perhaps most burdensome, an altered sense of self and inherent worth. Dignity has been defined in terms of being worthy of honour, respect, or esteem. Patients with a fractured sense of dignity not only felt their appearance had deteriorated, but—in the face of increasing neediness and dependency—reported a sense of being regarded as less worthy of respect or esteem.[25]

Thus, patients associate dignity with concepts such as respect and esteem, presumably including self-respect and self-esteem, whereas they experience its opposite—indignity—as degrading, shameful, or embarrassing.[26] These conceptual connections fit well under the primary *OED* definition of "dignity" as "the quality of being worthy or honourable." Abstractly speaking, a person's dignity seems to be a matter of assurance of her fully human status, both in her own eyes and in the eyes of others. Dignity is maintained when one can face others with pride and with confidence of being worthy of their respect; it is lost or impaired when being seen by others occasions feelings of shame, inferiority, or embarrassment. The element of degradation that is implicated in indignity seems a matter of feeling demoted or diminished from a higher standing to a lower, perhaps from the status of a fully functioning person to something lesser—an infant, for example, or even a thing.

This notion of indignity, understood in terms of debasement or dehumanization, plays a prominent role in contexts other than end-of-life care.

---

[25] Chochinov et al., "Dignity and the Terminally Ill," 2029.

[26] The same idea was voiced in another study, in which dignity was taken to mean "leaving a person with a body that he/she must not be ashamed of, or disgusted with"; Sabrina Cipolletta and Nadia Oprandi, "What Is a Good Death? Health Care Professionals' Narrations on End-of-Life Care," *Death Studies* 38, no. 1 (2014): 20–27, 24. Christopher Hitchens put the point nicely when, confronted by his own imminent demise due to cancer of the esophagus, he was asked whether he feared death: "No. I'm not afraid of being dead. . . . I'm afraid of a sordid death. I'm afraid that I will die in an ugly or squalid way, and cancer can be very vigorous in that respect" (interview with Jeremy Paxman for BBC Two's *Newsnight*, originally broadcast November 29, 2010).

Discussions of torture, for instance, typically stress the ways in which its badness, or wrongness, involves more than just the pain it inflicts. Torture does not just hurt its victim but also degrades or humiliates him or her.[27] In his treatment of torture—and of so-called cruel, inhuman, and degrading treatment—David Luban has emphasized this dimension of humiliation.[28] Torturers often add humiliation to pain by techniques such as stripping victims naked or sexually assaulting them. But the very experience of undergoing torture is humiliating in a more profound sense because the victim is utterly subordinated to the will of the torturer, never knowing when he or she might be subjected to even worse treatment. The humiliation aspect also emerges clearly in the infamous Abu Ghraib photographs. In Luban's words,

> They show terrified, naked detainees warding off attack dogs with their hands; shackled to the furniture in painful stress positions with women's underpants over their faces; led around on dog leashes; and standing naked in front of a leering female soldier. . . . The more lurid photos depict naked men piled in pyramids or smeared from head to toe in feces, or forced to urinate in each other's mouths.[29]

Luban concludes, "I trust that nobody will deny the obvious—that the evil depicted in these photographs is the humiliation and degradation of these detainees, the all-out assault on their human dignity." For Luban, therefore, "respecting human dignity means something quite down to earth: It means not humiliating people."[30]

Humiliation, of course, belongs to the same family of indignities as "the feeling of being degraded, ashamed, or embarrassed" reported by patients in the Chochinov study. The torture case serves as a reminder of how the experience of extreme pain can itself be degrading or humiliating if it is felt to be beyond one's control, either because it cannot be relieved or because its relief is subject to another's will. But it is easy to think of other conditions, perhaps especially likely at the end of life, that hospitalized patients might experience as humiliating, including being cathetered or

---

[27] See David Sussman, "What's Wrong with Torture?" *Philosophy & Public Affairs* 33, no. 1 (2005): 1–33. Other forms of treatment whose harmfulness takes the distinctive form of degrading or humiliating the victim include slavery, forced labor, internment in a concentration or death camp, rape, and discrimination.

[28] Luban, "Human Dignity, Humiliation, and Torture."

[29] Luban, "Human Dignity, Humiliation, and Torture," 221–222.

[30] Luban, "Human Dignity, Humiliation, and Torture," 214.

diapered for the excretion of body waste, being unable to clean or groom themselves, having their bodies exposed to the view of passing strangers, and being hooked up to an array of wires and tubes.

Jeremy Waldron has also invoked the notion of dignity in order to explicate what he regards as the harm done to minorities by hate speech.[31] For Waldron, dignity is a normative status: "A person's entitlement to be regarded as a member of society in good standing, as someone whose membership of a minority group does not disqualify him or her from ordinary social interaction."[32] For minorities, dignity requires acceptance by one's fellow citizens as belonging, recognition by them as a social equal, as well as the "*assurance* that one will be dealt with on this basis."[33] Waldron contends that dignity in this sense—as equal social standing plus the assurance of that standing—"is what hate speech attacks, and . . . what laws suppressing hate speech aim to protect."[34] Hate messages, he argues, are meant to warn members of their target minorities:

> Don't be fooled into thinking that you are welcome here. The society around you may seem hospitable and nondiscriminatory, but the truth is that you are not wanted, and you and your families will be shunned, excluded, beaten, and driven out, whenever we can get away with it. We may have to keep a low profile right now. But don't get too comfortable. Remember what has happened to you and your kind in the past. Be afraid.[35]

Waldron's analysis of dignity is, of course, fitted for his particular purposes in defending hate speech laws. But it does succeed in capturing the core idea of dignity as a kind of status or standing, assaults on which aim to degrade or debase the person or group into something less worthy of consideration and respect.

If we accept this broad characterization of indignity in terms of degradation or debasement, then it is possible to understand why the concept of dignity plays such a prominent role for dying patients and for their advocates. "Death with dignity" is not just a redescription of a good death, for that would empty the notion of all meaning. Instead, dignity is a convenient vehicle for collecting together many of the good-making features of a good death. This fact is perhaps best appreciated in the negative: Many, if

---

[31] Waldron, *The Harm in Hate Speech.*
[32] Waldron, *The Harm in Hate Speech*, 105.
[33] Waldron, *The Harm in Hate Speech*, 85.
[34] Waldron, *The Harm in Hate Speech*, 105.
[35] Waldron, *The Harm in Hate Speech*, 10.

not all, of the conditions that patients regard as compromising the quality of their dying they also experience as indignities.[36]

Thus far, the evidence concerning the ingredients of a dignified death has come from the patients themselves or from those closely connected to the patients (i.e., family, caregivers, and health care practitioners). On the negative side, what patients regard as indignities at the end of life seems a matter of what leaves them feeling "degraded, ashamed, or embarrassed." This raises the question of whether dignity and indignity are basically subjective notions, rooted in a patient's personal response to an external situation or form of treatment. The connection between indignity and humiliation seems to lend support to this interpretation. After all, the same set of circumstances might be experienced as humiliating by one person but not by another.[37] Consider, for instance, the fact of being dependent on others for intimate functions such as bathing and toileting. Some people—call them the "ruggedly independent"—have been accustomed to being in charge of their own personal care throughout their lives and experience the loss of that independence as acutely demeaning or degrading. For them, being reduced to the status of an infant demotes them below their own personal level of respectability, diminishing their self-esteem. Others, however, may experience this transition to dependence quite differently, perhaps as a sign of the love or commitment of those closest to them. Rather than feeling ashamed or humiliated, they may feel accepted and affirmed by the efforts that others are willing to make on their behalf. If so, then in this situation indignity seems to consist entirely in the subjective response of the recipient of care.

This subjectivizing of dignity and indignity is tempting, but it may be a little too extreme. In his treatment of dignity, for the purposes of explicating the harms of hate speech, Jeremy Waldron resists it. His particular burden is to identify the boundary between dignity, whose protection by law he deems legitimate, and offense, whose protection would be illegitimate. Waldron states,

---

[36] For the very considerable overlap between indignities and the factors that threaten a good death (or a good dying), see Karen E. Steinhauser et al., "In Search of a Good Death: Observations of Patients, Families, and Providers," *Annals of Internal Medicine* 132, no. 10 (2000): 825–832; Cipolletta and Oprandi, "What Is a Good Death?"

[37] In the mid-1990s, the mayor of a small French town banned the practice of "dwarf-tossing" in bars and clubs on the ground that it was degrading to the participants. However, one of the dwarves in question argued against the ban, saying that the competitions did not violate his dignity because he freely chose to take part in them and that they provided him with a job and a sense of self-worth. Despite his protestations, the French courts upheld the ban on grounds of human dignity. Smith, *End-of-Life Decisions in Medical Care*, 141.

The distinction is in large part between objective or social aspects of a person's standing in society, on the one hand, and subjective aspects of feeling, including hurt, shock, and anger, on the other. A person's dignity or reputation has to do with how things are with respect to them in society, not with how things feel to them.[38]

Waldron would undoubtedly want to draw the same distinction between dignity—or better, indignity—and feelings of shame, embarrassment, or humiliation. On his view, your dignity can be compromised—you can be subjected to an indignity—even if you do not experience it as such. And he seems to want to ground this possibility in the fact that a person's dignity has to do not only with her standing in her own eyes—her self-esteem—but also with the esteem in which she is held by others. If the latter can be lowered without the former—that is, without the subject feeling debased or degraded—then dignity and indignity cannot be purely subjective notions.

David Luban's identification of dignity with non-humiliation would seem to invite the subjective interpretation. Surely humiliation is a feeling, a subjective response to a perceived indignity. But Luban thinks otherwise. His burden is to explain how dignity can serve as the ground of universal human rights when feelings of humiliation might be culturally specific, with members of different cultures responding in very different ways to the same situations or forms of treatment. In order to meet this burden, he must treat humiliation itself as more than a subjective response. He attempts to persuade through a thought experiment:

A student drinks too much at a party and passes out. Some malicious wise-acres proceed to undress her and exhibit her naked body to everyone at the party—friends, acquaintances, dorm-mates, and strangers. Then they put her clothes back on, and when she wakes up and sobers up, nobody tells her what happened. In my view, the most natural and correct thing to say is that she has been humiliated—even if she never finds out and never has any subjective experience of humiliation.[39]

"In much the same way," Luban continues, "I believe that cultural practices of human subordination may be objectively humiliating, even though

---

[38] Waldron, *The Harm in Hate Speech*, 106.
[39] Luban, "Human Dignity, Humiliation, and Torture," 219.

participants in the practice are so used to it that it does not cause them psychological pain."[40]

Luban's thought experiment is compelling because it is easy to imagine a similar scenario involving an unconscious patient. Just such a scenario was part of the narrative line in the film *Kill Bill: Vol. 1*, in which the central character, known only as The Bride, spends four years in hospital in a coma after being shot in the head. During that time, an orderly has been charging his male friends for the opportunity to view her body and have sex with her. It being a Tarantino film, The Bride of course exacts bloody revenge once she awakes and realizes what has been going on. But, as Luban suggests, it seems entirely natural and correct to say that she has been subjected to a humiliation—an indignity—whether or not she ever finds out.

Both Waldron and Luban trade on the social or relational aspect of dignity, the extent to which it depends on the esteem in which others hold us. For our purposes, however, it is unnecessary to resolve this subjective/ objective dialectic definitively. The evidence from the Chochinov study shows that many patients feel degraded, ashamed, or embarrassed by such conditions as loss of autonomy or independence, deterioration in personal appearance, the need for assistance with intimate functions, and the experience of uncontrolled pain. It does not really matter if there are outliers who are content to have others in charge or do not care about their appearance or are stoical about pain. The statistically normal patient responses to these conditions give us ample reason to structure end-of-life care so as to avoid them as much as possible for all patients or to ensure that, when they become inevitable, we listen carefully to the ways in which particular patients experience them. The fact that there will be variations in those responses and experiences does not really matter. What matters is providing patients with the full range of options, including a physician-assisted death, for dealing with the dying process when they have come to find it an assault on their dignity.

The time has come to recap the direction of this discussion. Many have noted the chameleon-like ability of dignity to turn up on both the pro-choice side and the anti-choice side of the assisted death debate. I began by distinguishing the thin Kantian conception of dignity employed by anti-choice theorists such as David Velleman, in which dignity is nothing but the label for a particular kind of value or worth alleged to be inherent in

---

[40] Luban, "Human Dignity, Humiliation, and Torture," 219.

human beings (or persons)—a value weighty enough to have lexical priority over their interests or well-being. I then contrasted this with the thick conception available to the pro-choice side, in which dignity is a matter of maintaining a standard of respectability or self-esteem and in which indignities comprise a range of conditions and experiences that patients find debasing or degrading. What these two conceptions of dignity have in common is the notion of having a high-level status or importance, captured in the *OED* definition as "the quality of being worthy or honourable"; that is why they are two conceptions of the same abstract concept.

I am in no position to legislate terminology or to forbid one side of the debate or the other to strengthen its case with the considerable rhetorical force of the concept of dignity. However, I conclude by offering two reasons for preferring the thick conception to the thin. One is simply the fact that it is thick. The empirical content packed into thick notions makes them more informative than thin ones and therefore less replaceable. The thin Kantian notion of dignity can be replaced without loss by the notion of value or worth, as is often done in translations of the relevant passage from the *Groundwork*. But the thick notion has no equivalent or substitute. We can, of course, convey its content by other means, employing positive cognates such as self-esteem or self-respect or negative ones such as degradation, debasement, shame, and humiliation. But the thick conception serves as an efficient means of conveying that content and thus of pointing us to what seem to be normatively germane dimensions of end-of-life care— dimensions that help to make a case for the kind of patient control of the dying process that can be afforded by access to physician-assisted death.

My second reason for siding with the thick conception looks not to the content of speech but to the speakers. The thin conception is the property of philosophers such as Velleman who use it to construct a peculiarly Kantian case for their anti-choice stance. By contrast, as the empirical evidence has shown, the thick conception belongs to those who are immersed in the daily practice of end-of-life care: practitioners, families, and, above all, patients. Philosophers will never lack the opportunity to articulate their arguments and make their interventions into the public debate. But the voices of those whose interests are most at stake in that debate are often lost. Political scientists distinguish between two kinds of interest groups. Compact groups are centralized, organized, and effective at getting their message across in the public forum. Where the assisted death debate is concerned, the Catholic Church is the ultimate compact interest group. Diffuse groups, by contrast, are scattered and unorganized, and their voices are weak and easy to overlook or ignore. In the assisted death debate, dying patients—distributed across hospitals, nursing homes, and palliative care institutions—are the ultimate diffuse group. Their interests can to a certain extent be represented by right-to-die organizations or by prominent public spokespersons, but by virtue of their situation, they are rarely in a position to speak effectively for themselves.[41] I think that it is important for their voices to be heard. If they choose to frame their message in the language of dignity, as it is entirely appropriate that they should, then we should ensure that that language is taken seriously.

Thus, although I cannot legislate language for others, I can do so for myself. Henceforth, I will refuse to dignify the Kantian anti-choice position by characterizing it in terms of dignity, meeting it instead on the landscape of inherent value or worth. And I will make more and better room for dignity on my side of the debate. At the outset, I said that I am not the ideal spokesperson for the language of dignity because I managed to largely overlook it in making a case for the ethics and legality of assisted death. I now think that was a mistake, and were I to undertake the same task again, I would accord dignity considerably more attention.

However, it is only fair to say as well that the additional attention would not really change anything of importance for the case I continue to want to make. As I indicated previously, I built that case around the twin values of autonomy and well-being. In the course of exploring the thick conception of dignity, we have learned much about its relationship to these two values. One condition that patients report as degrading—as an indignity—is loss of control over the course of their own health care. Loss of autonomy matters in its own right, but it matters even more if it is the source for patients of shame and humiliation. This suggests that autonomy and well-being are themselves interconnected: Patients typically experience a loss of the former as a decline in the latter, as something that makes their dying process go worse for them by causing them feelings of indignity. Appeals to dignity thus flesh out what is at stake for patients in terms of their autonomy and well-being, but they do not introduce any factors that fall outside the limits of these values.

On the other hand, the language of dignity is unlikely to capture everything that patients find to compromise their dying process. Consider intractable pain, for example. Some patients—fortunately, a small

---

[41] Patients with progressive neurodegenerative disorders such as amyotrophic lateral sclerosis have been a conspicuous exception in both Canada and the United Kingdom because the slow progress of their illnesses has provided them with the time to become public figures. But most patients who opt for a physician-assisted death, where it is available, are suffering from end-stage cancer. Their condition usually affords them little opportunity for organizing or campaigning.

minority—experience intolerable pain that cannot be relieved by any measure short of deep unconsciousness or death. One thing we have learned is that the experience of such pain can itself be an indignity, so here again the language of dignity helps to illuminate what is at stake for such patients. But not all patients may experience pain as a blow to their self-esteem; for them, it might just be something they wish to be rid of. In their case, intractable pain remains an evil, an experience incompatible with a good death, regardless of whether it is also an indignity. The language of dignity can capture much of what matters to patients in the dying process and much of what may motivate them to seek an assisted death, but it cannot capture all of it. We lose important information as well if we simply equate a good death with a dignified death.

CHAPTER 5 | Death with Dignity
| *A Dangerous Euphemism*

CHRISTOPHER KACZOR AND ROBERT P. GEORGE

ADVOCATES OF PHYSICIAN-ASSISTED suicide and euthanasia sometimes speak of "death with dignity" and the "right to die with dignity." In a certain sense, no one's right to die can ever be jeopardized because everyone's death is a certainty that no law, no political institution, and no culture can prevent. The "right" to die, in that sense, has no greater need of legal and ethical defense than the right to be subject to gravity. What is at issue is not a right to die but, rather, a right to kill—the legal or moral right to intentionally end someone's life. Not dying (considered as something that inevitably happens), but euthanasia (considered as killing someone putatively for their own good) is the issue. We mean by "euthanasia" or "mercy killing" the intentional killing of a human being, either as a means to an end other than making the person in question dead or as an end in itself, undertaken with the motivation of benefiting the one who is killed. The choice to kill may be carried out as either active euthanasia, which is an intentional *act* such as injecting someone with poison, or passive euthanasia, which is an intentional *omission* aimed at producing death by, for example, withholding the nutrition and hydration necessary for survival. Some forms of intentionally killing the sick, disabled, or suffering are not undertaken for the sake of the sick, disabled, or suffering. These killings are undertaken to help other people, such those who are tired of caring for the needy, those who wish to save money that would otherwise be spent on their care, or those who look to obtain organs for transplantation. Properly speaking, these cases are not of euthanasia, for in these cases one person is killed for the sake of benefiting another person or other people. We confine our discussion to euthanasia in the sense of intentional killing undertaken for the sake of the one killed rather than intentional killing of one person in hopes of aiding others.

The right to intentionally kill an individual is sometimes justified by invoking "dignity." Like other words and concepts central to ethical discourse, such as "rights" and "autonomy," "dignity" is used in a variety of senses. In its root etymology, "dignity" is connected to worth and value. In its contemporary usage, we can distinguish four senses of the term, namely dignity as flourishing, dignity as attributed, dignity as intrinsic worth, and dignity as equivalent to or at least expressing autonomy.[1] We argue that none of these four senses of dignity justify intentional killing.

Dignity as flourishing is a life lived enjoying basic human goods. A flourishing human life includes acting in ways that are upright, virtuous, and reasonable. So, the person who habitually acts with personal integrity has dignity as flourishing in that respect. Sulmasy puts it as follows:

> Thus, dignity is sometimes used to refer to a state of virtue—a state of affairs in which a human being habitually acts in ways that expresses the intrinsic value of the human. We say, for instance, that so-and-so faced a particularly trying situation with dignity. This use of the word is not purely attributed, since it depends upon some objective conception of human excellence. Nonetheless, the value to which this use of the word refers is not intrinsic, since it depends upon a prior understanding of the intrinsic value of the human.[2]

Dignity as flourishing need not be limited simply to flourishing brought about by reasonable choices. Any human being enjoying basic human goods such as knowledge, friendship, life, and health may be said to enjoy dignity as flourishing with respect to those goods. Thus, a human being suffering from cancer may lack dignity as flourishing inasmuch as her health is

---

[1] For a more in-depth explanation of the first three senses of the term, see Daniel P. Sulmasy, "Dignity and Bioethics: History, Theory, and Selected Applications," in *Human Dignity and Bioethics: Essays Commissioned by the President's Council on Bioethics*, edited by Adam Schulman, Edmund D. Pellegrino, and Thomas W. Merrill (Washington, DC: US Independent Agencies and Commissions, 2008), 469–501. The fourth sense of the term is suggested by Ruth Macklin, who holds that dignity can be reduced to respect for autonomy. See Ruth Macklin, "Dignity Is a Useless Concept," *British Medical Journal* 327 (2003): 1419–1420.
[2] Sulmasy, "Dignity and Bioethics," 473.

failing but enjoy dignity as flourishing in another respect inasmuch as she faces her declining health with equanimity and courageous resolve.

Dignity as attributed can be defined as worth, honor, and respect bestowed upon an individual by the community or by individual choice. As Daniel Sulmasy states,

> By attributed dignity, I mean that worth or value that human beings confer upon others by acts of attribution. The act of conferring this worth or value may be accomplished individually or communally, but it always involves a choice. Attributed dignity is, in a sense, created. It constitutes a conventional form of value. Thus, we attribute worth or value to those we consider to be dignitaries, those we admire, those who carry themselves in a particular way, or those who have certain talents, skills, or powers. We can even attribute worth or value to ourselves using this word.[3]

The President of the United States getting a twenty-one gun salute, the scholar getting hooded *honoris causa*, and the Olympic champion receiving the gold medal enjoy attributed dignity. The contrary of dignity as attributed is dishonoring, shaming, and even torturing particular people because they are viewed as deserving such treatment.

By contrast, intrinsic dignity does not depend on human choice but, rather, on the inherent nature of the individual in question. Intrinsic dignity follows from the nature of the individual and remains as long as the individual continues to exist. Sulmasy describes it as follows:

> By intrinsic dignity, I mean that worth or value that people have simply because they are human, not by virtue of any social standing, ability to evoke admiration, or any particular set of talents, skills, or powers. Intrinsic dignity is the value that human beings have simply by virtue of the fact that they are human beings. Thus we say that racism is an offense against human dignity. Used this way, dignity designates a value not conferred or created by human choices, individual or collective, but is prior to human attribution.[4]

We might also call this endowment dignity because it is linked to the nature of the individual and is not achieved by the individual or given to the individual by others. We have endowment dignity or intrinsic dignity in virtue of our humanity, in virtue of our rational nature.

---

[3] Sulmasy, "Dignity and Bioethics," 473.
[4] Sulmasy, "Dignity and Bioethics," 473.

Finally, dignity may be understood as reducible to autonomy. Individuals have dignity if and only if they have the capacity to choose autonomously. To respect someone's dignity is nothing more than respecting someone's autonomy. As Ruth Macklin argues,

> "Dignity" seems to have no meaning beyond what is implied by the principle of medical ethics, respect for persons: the need to obtain voluntary, informed consent; the requirement to protect confidentiality; and the need to avoid discrimination and abusive practices. . . . Why, then, do so many articles and reports appeal to human dignity, as if it means something over and above respect for persons or for their autonomy? . . . Although the aetiology may remain a mystery, the diagnosis is clear. Dignity is a useless concept in medical ethics and can be eliminated without any loss of content.[5]

On Macklin's view, dignity does not do any important work in medical ethics beyond respect for persons. This claim that dignity is a useless concept has been criticized and defended elsewhere,[6] but we do not need to adjudicate that dispute for our purposes. One way, although arguably not the only way, to understand dignity is as a respect for the autonomy of persons. How, then, do these four senses of dignity relate to forms of mercy killing?

Euthanasia and Dignity as Flourishing

Dignity as flourishing involves both moral well-being and non-moral well-being. To flourish is to enjoy the basic human goods. Human flourishing in its various dimensions presupposes and necessarily involves the human being's continued existence. No individual can have a flourishing life unless that individual is alive. To flourish or fail to flourish qualifies the life. One cannot have a low or a high quality of life without being alive.

But perhaps dignity as flourishing can be used as a justification for euthanasia in the following way. Once flourishing falls beneath a certain threshold, a human being benefits from being killed. We might debate

---

[5] Macklin, "Dignity Is a Useless Concept," 1420.
[6] Perhaps the most well-known defense of Macklin's claim is Steven Pinker's "The Stupidity of Dignity," *The New Republic* 238, May 27, 2008. A critique of their views can be found in the first chapter of Christopher Kaczor, *A Defense of Dignity: Creating Life, Destroying Life, and Protecting the Rights of Conscience* (Notre Dame, Ind.: University of Notre Dame Press, 2013).

about what exactly that threshold is and whether crossing this threshold is sufficient for justifying euthanasia or whether autonomous consent is also necessary for justifying euthanasia. The intuition is that once dignity as flourishing has been irrevocably lost, it is better for the one in question no longer to exist at all.

Does illness, provided it is intense enough, make death beneficial? Imagine a sliding scale of human physical well-being. On one extreme, you find Olympic athletes in the flower of youth and the peak of strength, endurance, speed, and every dimension of healthy functioning. As you slide down the scale, this health functioning diminishes to increasingly lower levels until reaching the other extreme of the scale of human beings just on the verge of complete and irreversible loss of integrated organic functioning in all respects, namely death. The justification of euthanasia in terms of quality of life depends on the idea that intentional killing, even if authorized by the one killed, is ethically wrong and legally should be prohibited for the Olympic athlete. It is difficult to understand why somewhere along the scale of physical well-being intentionally killing human beings becomes not a harm inflicted upon them but, rather, a benefit to them. How can moving an individual further down the "scale" of physical dysfunction be a benefit to the individual? The further down the scale the individual goes, the worse off the individual is in terms of physical well-being. To kill an individual is to completely destroy the physical well-being of the individual. Killing an individual can never be a benefit to an individual. Benefits make an individual in some respect better off than the individual was prior to receiving the benefit. Intention killing, by contrast, does not make the individual killed better off but, rather, makes the individual nonexistent.

Euthanasia and Dignity as Attributed

At first glance, dignity as attributed has little to do with euthanasia. No one views mercy killing as an honor bestowed because of outstanding achievement in service of the public good. Nor is the justification for mercy killing the imposition of a kind of dishonor upon those at the end of life that they deserve to die because of some bad action that they have done. Euthanasia is not capital punishment.

Dignity as attributed can be used to justify euthanasia in that those who are intentionally killed either no longer have or soon will no longer have any value. If human worth is understood simply as attributed, then it depends on the judgment and choice of human beings. Just as we can celebrate and honor certain kinds of people, we can denigrate and dishonor other kinds of people. We may, therefore, judge that a certain class of people—for instance, those in the last six months of life or those who are enduring grave physical or mental suffering—do not have lives worth living. If certain kinds of human beings, such as those suffering or unconscious at the end of life, have no value, there is no disvalue in killing them, aside perhaps from circumstantial considerations.

Is it true that such human beings have no value? Consider a woman in a hospital in a persistent vegetative state who will soon be dying. Just after midnight, a janitor enters her room and has sexual intercourse with her. Everyone recognizes that this woman would be wronged and her basic rights violated because it is always wrong to have sexual intercourse with someone without that person's consent (i.e., to rape someone). But this intuition presupposes that she still has basic rights—that she is still someone who can be morally wronged. In other words, she still has value as a moral subject, despite her grave disability and imminent death.

Dignity as attribution can only justify euthanasia if we assume that human beings do not have intrinsic dignity. We might fail to value something that is in fact quite valuable, such as mistakenly thinking a painting is a knock-off when it is an actual work by Rembrandt. So, too, if we classify the gravely disabled as not having value and worth, if we deny them dignity of attribution in a basic sense, we may be making a serious mistaken. Thus, the case for euthanasia based on dignity of attribution depends on a denial of intrinsic dignity to some class of human individuals. For if human beings have intrinsic dignity, there is no human condition for which a basic dignity of attribution is not the proper response. Not every professor deserves an honorary doctorate; however, if dignity is intrinsic, every person deserves to be respected, even if the individual in question is suffering, at the end of life, or seriously disabled mentally and physically.

Of course, the suffering person may view herself as lacking any dignity. She may think that she currently is or will soon be worthless, and therefore that death is preferable to continuing to exist in her worthless condition. But it is certainly possible that an individual's self-evaluation is mistaken. The anorexic believes she is too fat and may seek help in losing weight. The severely depressed person may think that not only his life but also the lives of all human being lack any meaning, purpose, or significance. If human beings have intrinsic value, then an individual human being may be mistaken in denying his or her own worth.

Another way dignity as attributed may be used to justify euthanasia is by appeal to respect for choices. We acknowledge and realize the dignity of another as attributed by various means, such as by providing honors to them, by giving them words of praise, and by granting them social status. Dignity is also attributed when we recognize, accept, and respect the choices of others. In so doing, we treat another person, specifically the person as the source of free and autonomous choice, as having value. So, in cases of voluntary euthanasia as well as physician-assisted suicide, when choices to die are made autonomously, dignity as attributed leads to an acceptance of such decisions as a way of recognizing and reaffirming the worth of the agent as freely choosing his or her own way of dying. To respect other people, we must also respect their own autonomous choices, including their choice to die in the way that they choose.

Although dignity as attributed might be invoked to justify euthanasia or physician-assisted suicide, this justification is problematic. We should recognize and attribute dignity to others in ways that are fitting and responsible. But attributed dignity does not require accepting and respecting all the choices of others, no matter what these choices may be. An autonomous choice can also be selfish, stupid, self-contradictory, irrational, and immoral. We can and should always respect the person who is choosing, but we cannot and should not respect every choice that is made. The choice of the segregationist to exclude African Americans from full legal protection and the choice of the advocate of equality to include all human beings in full legal protection cannot consistently both be respected.

In the case of euthanasia, the full legal protection of all human beings is at stake. Laws allowing euthanasia carve out an exception to the equal protection of the lives of all members of the community, legalizing some cases of intentional killing. Legally permitting euthanasia implies that the vast majority of people's lives are worth fully protecting, but a small minority of people's lives (those who are suffering or nearing death) do not merit the same protection, and so they may be intentionally killed.

Even advocates of euthanasia do not hold that respect for the decisions of others alone requires acceptance of euthanasia. The legalization and/or the ethical permissibility is characteristically said to depend on not just an individual's choice but also other conditions, such as intense suffering, lack of mental illness, or an incurable disease. These qualifications limiting euthanasia may arise from a recognition that political conditions would not allow euthanasia at any time or for any reason. But part of the reason such a policy is so politically unpalatable is that important goods, such as protecting the vulnerable, would be jeopardized by such a law.

Another way in which dignity of attribution could be used to justify intentional mercy killing might be seen by way of analogy. A customary way of honoring a tattered US flag in the United States is to burn it. The rationale behind this practice is that it somehow dishonors what the flag represents to allow it to continue to fly when its condition has significantly deteriorated. In like manner, we intentionally kill an individual who is significantly deteriorating as a way of attributing dignity to the individual. We show dignity as attributed to deteriorating human beings at the end of life by no longer allowing them to continue in their deteriorated condition.

But we honor people by giving them something that is good. It is not honoring but, rather, dishonoring people to intentionally inflict evil upon them. To "honor" people by intentionally destroying their knowledge, their capacity to play, their friendships, or their appreciation of the beautiful is not to honor them at all but, rather, to harm them.

So the question about whether we can honor people by killing them depends in part on whether death is something good or evil for a human being. Like knowledge and friendship, to be alive is intrinsically good for a human being. Indeed, to be a human person necessarily involves being alive, for without life only a corpse remains. We are human beings, living organisms of a particular species. If we have intrinsic value, then these living organisms have intrinsic value. If we are intrinsically valuable, our lives (which are nothing other than ourselves as bodily) have intrinsic value. Death destroys the human being and so does not benefit a human being in any way. Yes, death may also lead to an end of suffering, but that does not mean that death itself is good. Good can come from evil and evil can rise from good without good being evil or evil being good. If someone is kidnapped and escapes, such a person may experience what positive psychologists call post-traumatic growth. The victim of the kidnapping may emerge more altruistic, patient, and virtuous. But this growth does not mean that kidnapping was not really evil.

Critics may respond that body–self dualism provides an alternative to the view that "we are human beings." According to body–self dualism, "we" are not properly speaking rational animals, organisms of a particular species; rather, "we" are our thoughts, beliefs, desires, and self-awareness. On this view, "we" may be intrinsically valuable, but our bodies are just akin to vehicles in which what is truly "us" (our thoughts, beliefs, desires, etc.) is located. "We" are intrinsically valuable persons, but our bodies are merely animal organisms that "we" inhabit (or are in some mysterious way associated with).

In *Body–Self Dualism in Contemporary Ethics and Politics*, one of the co-authors (RPG) provides reason to reject body–self dualism.[7] One consideration against body–self dualism arises from cases of multiple personality disorder. Suppose an individual human being has two independent sets of beliefs, desires, goals, and memories. This one human being is Dr. Jekyll and also Mr. Hyde. Now suppose a psychiatrist cures the multiple personality disorder, eliminating the Mr. Hyde set of memories, beliefs, and desires. Has the psychiatrist done an act of compassionate healing for which she deserves praise? Or should the psychiatrist be blamed for "destroying a person" and be subject to criminal prosecution for murder? If curing multiple personality disorder is praiseworthy rather than deserving of punishment, then "we" as valuable beings are not really constituted by our thoughts, beliefs, and desires rather than by a bodily human being.

Is burning the flag to honor the country analogous to euthanasia? The key difference is that the flag is just a symbol of the United States. It is a sign of the thing that is getting honored, not the actual thing itself. If the United States fell on hard times, economic collapse and political chaos, it would hardly be honoring the country to destroy whatever good it had left.

Euthanasia and Dignity as Intrinsic Worth

Sulmasy holds that dignity as intrinsic worth undergirds the other senses of dignity. Immanuel Kant provided the classic case against euthanasia and suicide in the *Grounding for the Metaphysics of Morals*. Kant writes,

> [If a person] destroys himself in order to escape from a difficult situation, then he is making use of his person merely as a means so as to maintain a tolerable condition till the end of his life. Man, however, is not a thing and hence is not something to be used merely as a means. He must in all his actions always be regarded as an end in himself. Therefore, I cannot dispose of man in my own person by mutilating, damaging, or killing him.[8]

Human persons have intrinsic dignity unlike things, which have a price. Mere things may be used, abused, or even destroyed for the sake of some other end. But human beings must always be respected as ends in

---

[7] See Patrick Lee and Robert P. George, *Body–Self Dualism in Contemporary Ethics and Politics* (New York: Cambridge University Press, 2007).

[8] Immanuel Kant, *Grounding for the Metaphysics of Morals*, trans. James W. Ellington, 3rd ed. (Indianapolis, Ind.: Hackett, 1993), 36.

themselves and may never be used simply as a means, killed, or maimed for some other end.

On this view, the value of a human being does not depend on whether the individual is experiencing pleasure, pain, or nothing at all. Human beings do not have value because of what they are experiencing but because of who they are. Indeed, we care about what human beings experience precisely because we care about human beings. If human beings themselves lack value, then why should we care about what human beings experience? The slave holder does not care about the slave and therefore is indifferent to the suffering of the slave.

Kant's insight might be reformulated. The basic human goods provide the ultimate reasons for action. These basic goods—such as knowledge, health, life, and friendship—are intrinsic goods rather than merely instrumental goods, such as money, prestige, and power. But to kill a human being in order to attain some other end is to reduce an intrinsic good to the status of a merely instrumental good. To act in this way is to confuse what is merely a means with what is an end in itself. It is to act unreasonably and immorally.

Euthanasia may be undertaken with various goals in mind: to end suffering, to respect a decision, to save money, or to escape from a hopeless situation. But whatever motivates the choice to intentionally kill, the person (in his or her bodily existence) is destroyed—is used up as it were in order to attain this other state of affairs.

The view that euthanasia is impermissible does not entail that all treatments that extend life must always be used regardless of circumstances. To say that every human person has intrinsic worth is not to claim that every treatment offered to a human person has intrinsic worth. In fact, some treatments are more burdensome than beneficial. If a particular treatment is painful, costly, and difficult to administer, this treatment may not be worthwhile for a particular patient. If the burdens of a particular treatment are substantial and the benefits of the treatment not as significant, then the treatment may be refused or discontinued. The proper judgment is not about whether the *person* is worthwhile but, rather, whether the *treatment* is worthwhile.[9]

Is there are gap between affirming the value of all persons and affirming that the lives of all persons are valuable? Could we not claim that all persons are valuable but that the biological lives of persons

---

[9] For more on this distinction, see Chapter 1 of John Keown, *The Law and Ethics of Medicine: Essays on the Inviolability of Human Life* (New York: Oxford University Press, 2012).

have value if and only if each person himself or herself values his or her life?

Such questions presuppose a body–self dualism in which the person is one thing but the person's bodily existence is another. Each individual person is intrinsically valuable, but the biological life of a person has only instrumental value.

But human persons are not souls trapped in bodies or functioning cerebral cortexes riding around in bodies as in a vehicle. A human being is a biological organism, and we are human beings.[10] So if we have value intrinsically, then human beings have value intrinsically and these biological organisms have value intrinsically.

Euthanasia and Dignity as Autonomy

Let us assume for the sake of argument that the moral import of "dignity" can be reduced to autonomy. Autonomy can be understood in a variety of ways.

For Kant, autonomy is the self-given law of practical reason, which is the same for all rational beings and binds all rational beings in having a duty to act only in accordance with the categorical imperative. Kant views every human being, indeed every rational being, as something "whose existence has in itself an absolute worth, something which is an end in itself."[11] This insight grounds the categorical imperative, which in one formulation obliges all rational beings to "act in such a way that you treat humanity, whether in your own person or in the person of another, always at the same time as an end and never simply as a means."[12] The duty imposed by the categorical imperative binds all rational agents "as the supreme limiting condition of every man's freedom of action."[13] To destroy an individual having absolute, unconditional worth for the sake of some (indeed, any) further end, even an otherwise legitimate end such as elimination of suffering, is not to act autonomously but, rather, in Kant's terms, to act heteronomously, to act against duty, to act unethically.

In a second sense, autonomy is understood to be exercised in any decision made by an individual who gives informed consent. So, if a patient

---

[10] For more on body–self dualism, see Lee and George, *Body–Self Dualism in Contemporary Ethics and Politics*.

[11] Kant, *Grounding for the Metaphysics of Morals*, 35.

[12] Kant, *Grounding for the Metaphysics of Morals*, 36.

[13] Kant, *Grounding for the Metaphysics of Morals*, 37.

understands the reality of his or her medical condition, appreciates the certain and/or likely ramifications of a potential choice, and after due reflection decides to execute a choice, then this choice is autonomous. Thus, if dignity is reduced to autonomy, and someone gives properly informed consent to physician-assisted suicide or voluntary euthanasia, then the value of human dignity supports physician-assisted suicide and voluntary euthanasia. In "The Philosopher's Brief," Ronald Dworkin et al. offer perhaps the most famous argument for euthanasia based on autonomy:

> Most of us see death—whatever we think will follow it—as the final act of life's drama, and we want that last act to reflect our own convictions, those we have tried to live by, not the convictions of others forced on us in our most vulnerable moment.[14]

Our choices determine the value of our lives and the circumstances of our deaths. So, respect for our human dignity entails a respect for our autonomy, and this leads to respect for the choices of assisted suicide and voluntary euthanasia. On this view, the value of autonomy trumps the value of human life.

A challenge to this view can be raised by considering the ground for ascribing value to autonomous choices. As Colin Bird notes, "Every human agent must attribute worth to his purposes . . . [because an agent] regards his purposes as good according to whatever criteria enter into his purposes."[15] If an agent views his or her goals as worthwhile, implicitly that agent is also affirming some sense of personal worth. The agent is the source of the action. If the action is valuable, the agent must also be valuable. Alan Gewirth puts the point as follows: "They are *his* purposes, and they are worth attaining because *he* is worth sustaining and fulfilling, so that he has what for him is a justified sense of his own worth."[16] The conclusion is that the "generic purposiveness" of rational action, just as such, "underlies the ascription of inherent dignity to all agents" (including oneself).[17] If this reasoning is correct, then intrinsic dignity undergirds dignity as autonomy. Why should we respect autonomy? The *autonomy* of a person matters only if the *person* matters. But if the person matters

---

[14] Ronald Dworkin et al., "Assisted Suicide: The Philosopher's Brief," *The New York Review of Books*, March 27, 1997: 41–47.

[15] Colin Bird, "Dignity as a Moral Concept," *Social Philosophy & Policy* 30, no. 1–2 (2013): 150–176.

[16] Alan Gewirth, *Self-Fulfillment* (Princeton, N.J.: Princeton University Press, 2009), 168–169.

[17] Gewirth, *Self-Fulfillment*, 169.

as an end in itself, as oriented to the goods that are the ultimate reason for action, then autonomy does not justify euthanasia.

Appeals to autonomy to justify euthanasia are often at cross-purposes with appeals to eliminating suffering to justify euthanasia. If it benefits a person at the end of life to be killed, why should this benefit be withheld from patients because the patients cannot consent to receive the benefit? Imagine two patients at the end of life. Both experience intolerable pain. One patient has the competence to give informed consent for euthanasia. The other patient not only suffers physical pain but also suffers from mental illness to such a degree that he cannot give informed consent to any medical treatment. If autonomy is necessary to justify euthanasia, the second patient—the worse-off patient—is not eligible for euthanasia.

On the other hand, if consent is not necessary for euthanasia, then the argument from dignity as autonomy is superfluous in the justification for intentional killing at the end of life. Indeed, justifications of euthanasia are often inconsistent in their appeals to autonomy. If there is no ethical difference between intentional killing and removing life support, because removing life support is permitted for the mentally ill and for minors lacking autonomy, then intentional killing of the mentally ill and minors should also be permitted. Of course, critics of euthanasia characteristically argue that there is an ethical difference between intentional killing and removing life support in cases in which the burdens of the treatment are not worth enduring or bearing in view of its comparatively meager benefits. But this difference is characteristically denied by advocates of the choice to kill. So, if removing life support and intentional killing are not ethically different, then consistency demands that whoever accepts removing life support for minor children and the mentally ill also accepts intentional killing of incompetent individuals. Thus, autonomy does no real work justifying euthanasia.

Perhaps dignity as autonomy is not a necessary condition for justifying mercy killing, but it is a sufficient condition. If a competent individual deems his or her life no longer worth living, then he or she may licitly receive voluntary euthanasia or a physician's (or other health care worker's) assistance in committing suicide. What makes a human being valuable is that the human being values continuing to exist, and if a human being no longer desires to continue to exist, then this human life no longer has value. It is wrong to kill an individual because that individual values his or her life. And if the individual does not value his or her life, then it is not wrong to kill the individual.

As John Keown notes, the claim that "a person's life has value only if the person values it" is vague, arbitrary, discriminatory, and dualistic.[18] The claim is vague because our desires are by nature vague, shifting, difficult to define, and sometimes growing in intensity and then shrinking in intensity. How can we all have fundamental equality as persons if our value as persons depends on the vagaries and shifting foundation of human desires? The claim that we have value because we value our own lives is arbitrary. As John Finnis notes,

> Why not pick out other features which characterize human nature in its flourishing—say linguistic articulacy, sense of humour, and/or friendship more deep, transparent, and supple than friendship between man and dog? Why not then call one or other or some set of these the capacity which, while it is enjoyed, makes us people and "entitles and individual to be considered a person"?[19]

The claim is discriminatory, for if an individual in his or her bodily existence is only valuable if he or she as a matter of subjective psychological fact happens to desire to continue to live, then some people who are depressed, mentally handicapped, severely intoxicated, or brainwashed to not value their own lives are excluded from equality in value with others in the human community. Finally, the claim that our value as human beings depends on our desires is implicitly dualistic, supposing that "we" (beings who can value) exist only when our desires begin to exist, as if our bodies were mere transporters of the reality of merely mental selves.

If autonomy is a sufficient justification for mercy killing, we have no reasoned justification for excluding non-suffering competent adults (or mature minors) from euthanasia. If competent people consider their own lives not worth living, on what basis should we exclude them from having a "right to die" just because they lack physical suffering or are not in the last stages of a terminal illness? People may consider their lives not worth living for a wide variety of reasons, such as the loss of a significant romantic relationship or frustrated life plans. You or I may not agree with such reasoning, but that fact is completely irrelevant, at least according to a purely subjective justification of euthanasia based on autonomy.

---

[18] John Keown, "A New Father for Law and Ethics of Medicine," in *Reason, Morality, and Law: The Philosophy of John Finnis*, edited by John Keown and Robert P. George (Oxford: Oxford University Press, 2013), 300.

[19] John Finnis, *Human Rights and Common Good. Collected Essays of John Finnis: Volume III* (Oxford: Oxford University Press, 2011), 226.

Conclusion

None of the four senses of dignity explored in this chapter—namely dignity as flourishing, dignity as attributed, dignity as intrinsic worth, and dignity as autonomy—provide a sound justification of euthanasia. "Death with dignity" and the "right to die with dignity" are dangerous euphemisms masking the reality of what is at issue in these cases, which is not precisely death or dying but, rather, intentional killing. Such euphemisms obscure the reality that all human persons are equal in fundamental dignity and that this basic value remains undiminished even at the end of life, even in the midst of suffering. The proper ethical response to human problems such as suffering is, if possible, to eliminate the problem, not to eliminate the human. The ethically proper legal response is to accord to every person within the jurisdiction fully and equally the law's fundamental protection against intentional killing.

SECTION 3 | Dignity and Disability

CHAPTER 6 | Physical Disability, Dignity, and Physician-Assisted Death

DAVID WASSERMAN

IN THIS CHAPTER, I consider the relevance of physical disability for dignity-based claims to physician assistance in dying (PAD). Because the loss of major bodily functions often accompanies terminal illness, physical disability is frequently adduced in justifying PAD, either to shorten a now-undignified life or to permit a "death with dignity."[1] But it is also invoked to claim indignity, and demand PAD, in circumstances in which death is not (otherwise) imminent. In jurisdictions that permit PAD in the face of "unbearable and irremediable suffering" (or words to that effect), the requisite suffering has been found to result from the indignity of severe physical disability. Even if it does not lead to unbearable suffering, such disability may also be regarded as sufficiently undignified to warrant PAD.

I argue that physical disability, however severe, provides no stronger dignity-based reason than other kinds of loss or misfortune for permitting PAD. My primary concern is with the use of physical disability as a paradigm of indignity in many standard arguments for PAD. This concern is well expressed by Katherina Heyer:

---

[1] A general issue, which I raise but do not pursue, concerns the distinction between endorsing (assisted) suicide as a means of simply minimizing the indignity of continued life and endorsing it as a means of restoring or achieving dignity. An individual or society may regard a condition or situation as undignified but hold that suicide is an inappropriate response, which may even compound the indignity. But an individual or society also can view suicide not merely as ending indignity but as restoring a lost dignity or as achieving a dignity the individual never previously had. Dignity restoration is suggested by the suicide of Othello, the Venetian general manipulated into killing his innocent wife. In stabbing himself as he once stabbed a Muslim who gravely insulted Venice, he restores his role as its protector and avenger. The achievement of greater dignity in death than in life is suggested by the postmortem on Macbeth (who died in battle, not by suicide): "Nothing in his life became him like the leaving it."

Proponents of [PAD] point to the loss of bodily autonomy that accompanies terminal illness that needs to be recovered by the assertion of autonomy over death. Yet this loss of bodily autonomy is a commonplace experience for people with disabilities, many of whom require daily personal assistance with the most private aspects of daily living.[2]

In denying that severe physical disability is paradigmatically or presumptively undignified, I do not argue against the extension of PAD to nonterminal cases. I merely argue that there is no principled basis for limiting the extension to individuals with a severe disease or disability.[3]

I proceed as follows. First, I briefly consider the role of physical disability in making the case for PAD in cases of terminal illness. I suggest that dignity-based claims in general have greater force in that context than in nonterminal cases but deny that physical disability has any special relevance for those claims. I then explore the role of physical disability in dignity-based claims to PAD in the absence of terminal illness, either in satisfying a standard of "unbearable and irremediable suffering" or as an independent ground for suicide. After raising a general problem with adducing indignity to claim such suffering, I examine the relevance of physical disability for indignity as an independent basis for PAD.

This inquiry, which takes up most of the chapter, makes use of three hypothetical cases in which PAD is sought on the grounds of profound indignity. I argue that there is no greater indignity in the case involving physical disability than in the other two cases, or, more generally, in cases of physical disability than other conditions. I then seek to fortify this intuitive judgment by considering three plausible approaches to human dignity developed in the recent literature, which, I argue, yield similar verdicts for all three cases.

Physical Disability and Dignity in Terminal Illness

Arguably, disability-based dignity considerations have a relevance in end-of-life contexts that they lack elsewhere. A person who loses speech, mobility, or sphincter control through terminal illness typically has little

---

[2] Katherina Heyer, "Rejecting Rights: The Disability Critique of Physician Assisted Suicide," in *Special Issue Social Movements/Legal Possibilities*, edited by Austin Sarat (Somerville, MA: Emerald Group, 2011), 77–112, 81.

[3] That restriction need not be justified in terms of (in)dignity. As I discuss later, some scholars argue for it on the dubious ground that PAD will count as a medical treatment if and only if it is offered in response to a medical condition.

opportunity to reconstruct her life without those functions. PAD gives her a way to repudiate physical losses and limitations to which her terminal condition gives her little or no opportunity to adapt. But a dying individual has no greater opportunity to adapt to other losses—of reputation, professional stature, fond hopes, or close companions. Of course, these losses are not associated with terminal illness, in contrast to the physical disabilities that accompany, and are often caused by, that illness. But even if they have a more contingent relationship to the dying process, those losses may equally contribute to the conviction that it is futile to briefly extend a life that has lost meaning or purpose and that affords little opportunity to regain it. Rather than justifying a special role for physical disability, this lack of opportunity suggests a distinct rationale for the restriction of PAD to terminal illness (possibly with an "unbearable suffering" exception)—not only because of the lesser risk of abuse but also because of the vanishing prospects for restorative or redemptive adaptation.

Although I have framed it in terms of dignity, this rationale for restricting PAD to terminal illness is quite different than the Kantian rationale suggested by David Velleman. For Velleman, it is not the lack of time and opportunity to give meaning or purpose to one's losses that may justify assisted suicide but, rather, the presence of pain so overwhelming that it destroys the source of worth or value in human life: "Pain that tyrannizes the patient . . . undermines his rational agency, by preventing him from choosing any ends for himself other than relief."[4] Such pain would be sufficient but not necessary to justify PAD on a rationale based on an irremediable loss of meaning or purpose. Someone with weeks to live who had lost almost all that she valued in life would be eligible for PAD on such a rationale. She would not, however, be eligible for PAD on Velleman's account if her rationality could be preserved by suitable pain management or psychological support.

Beyond Terminal Illness

Currently, most jurisdictions that permit PAD in the absence of terminal illness do so only in cases of unbearable and irremediable pain or suffering.[5] In those jurisdictions, claims of indignity are relevant only as evidence

---

[4] David Velleman, "A Right of Self-Termination?", *Ethics* 109, no. 3 (1999): 606–628, 618.
[5] See, for example, Udo Schüklenk et al., "End-of-Life Decision-Making in Canada: The Report by the Royal Society of Canada Expert Panel on End-of-Life Decision-Making," *Bioethics* 25, no. s1 (2011): 1–73.

of such suffering. But citing the contribution of indignity to unbearable suffering does not seem to offer the right kind of reason for a dignity-based claim to assistance. It requires the victim of indignity to make the same kind of claim as the victim of intense chronic pain or overwhelming grief: that her condition causes her a degree of suffering that she cannot bear or—more accurately—should not be expected to bear. But this claim distorts the moral force of dignity as a ground for suicide, assisted or not. The individual who seeks to end her life because of its indignity need not be seeking to end her suffering. Apart from her indignity, she may find her suffering tolerable or may not experience much suffering at all. There may be little correlation between the depth of an indignity and the magnitude of the suffering arising from it. Indeed, indignities do not even need to be experienced to count as harms or wrongs, e.g., the cruel ridicule of an individual who lacks the capacity to understand the insult. In contrast, suffering, however broadly defined, is a kind of experience; it makes no sense to talk about unexperienced suffering.

Even if serious indignities generally caused "unbearable and irremediable" suffering, honoring dignity-based claims because and to the extent that they did would involve taking something like Peter Strawson's "objective attitude" toward the victims of indignity.[6] It would treat them as the passive subjects of aversive feelings rather than the bearers of standards or norms from which, as they see it, they have fallen egregiously short. Because this concern is relevant to any dignity-based claim under an intolerable-suffering criterion, not just those arising from physical disabilities, I bracket it here and just assume that sufficiently deep indignity counts as unbearable suffering.

But this assumption changes the significance of the state authorization of assisted suicide in nonterminal cases. An unbearable-suffering criterion, like a terminal-illness criterion, can claim a compassionate if not strictly medical rationale. These rationales offer a kind of neutrality because they do not require the state to make controversial normative judgments about what makes a life go, or end, well or badly. Suffering, like terminal illness, is arguably something that can be assessed scientifically—there are reliable statistics for the latter and validated scales for the former. Admittedly, judgments about the legitimacy of the causes of suffering may distort its assessment—suffering from chronic illness or severe disability may be overestimated, whereas suffering from personal loss may be

---

[6] Peter Frederick Strawson, *Freedom and Resentment and Other Essays* (London: Routledge, 2008), 9.

underestimated. But there are presumably checks and correctives for such potential distortions.

In contrast, judging indignities on their own terms, and not in terms of their contribution to unbearable suffering, requires debatable, value-laden judgments about what counts as a deep or serious indignity and about whether assisted suicide would be indignity-mitigating or dignity-restoring. The state may not be able to avoid making such judgments. But if it makes them, it should get them right; in the case of physical disability, it is disturbingly likely to get them wrong. There is considerable evidence that physicians generally evaluate the quality of life of patients with disabilities as significantly lower than do the patients and their families.[7] Even when, as in requesting PAD, patients judge their quality of life to be very low, physicians are unlikely to provide a check on subjective judgments that, as I argue in the next section, may reflect a lack of social support as much as a loss of meaning or purpose.

Three Hypothetical Cases

Compare three individuals who request PAD on the basis of profound indignity, none of whom has a terminal or degenerative illness or intense, chronic physical pain:

1. A is a self-made billionaire, proud of her independence, shrewdness, and the respect and deference of her three sons. She decides to retire early and turn all her holdings over to her sons in equal shares. The older two effusively praise her decision; the youngest questions the wisdom of relinquishing control so early. Stung by his doubts, she disinherits him and divides his share between his brothers. Things go badly from the start. The two older sons keep their mother on a tight leash and a meager pension, and they condescendingly dismiss her financial advice. Humiliated by being treated as a nuisance and a burden, and disheartened by the defeat of a hostile takeover bid by her youngest son to restore her interests, she finds it worse than pointless, even pathetic, to go on.

---

[7] David Alan Klein, "Medical Disparagement of the Disability Experience: Empirical Evidence for the 'Expressivist Objection'," *AJOB Primary Research* 2, no. 2 (2011): 8–20; Carole J. Gill, "Health Professionals, Disability, and Assisted Suicide: An Examination of Relevant Empirical Evidence and Reply to Batavia," *Psychology, Public Policy and the Law* 6 (2000): 526–545; Saroj Saigal et al., "Differences in Preferences for Neonatal Outcomes among Health Care Professionals, Parents, and Adolescents," *JAMA* 281, no. 21 (1999): 1991–1997.

2. B is the highly respected long-term mayor of a small town, with a spotless reputation. At a convention of municipal officials in a large city, however, she gets drunk and hires an underage prostitute. At his apartment, he strips her, ties her up, and spanks her. He secretly videotapes their encounter. Even more unfortunately, she is spotted by a cyberjournalist as she leaves the apartment. He buys the prostitute's video and posts it online, where it goes viral. She is convicted of a sex offense, made to register as a sex offender, and forced to resign. Her spouse divorces her, and her friends shun her. During the next several years, she tries and fails to make a political comeback and to rehabilitate her reputation. Shamed and isolated, she finds it worse than pointless, even pathetic, to go on.

3. C is a mountaineer who gets tremendous personal satisfaction and professional recognition from her climbs. She trains almost obsessively but finds her routine rewarding, not confining. She avoids injury on her climbs but loses all four limbs to a rare disease. Initially, she expects to discover other rewarding pursuits, such as lecturing about her climbs or coaching aspiring mountaineers. But it does not happen. Those activities merely increase her longing for the first-hand experiences she can never have again, and she finds no satisfaction in other kinds of activity. She regards her present condition, in which she needs help with daily activities such as toileting, as shamefully dependent, a reproach to her past life of proud self-reliance and calculated risk-taking. It seems worse than pointless, even pathetic, to go on.

All three individuals have had their lives disrupted by events not fully within their control; all have failed to find a satisfactory alternative; all regard their present situation as deeply undignified. Their desire to end their lives is clearly rational, if not reasonable. Whether they should be granted PAD to end their lives, it does not seem that the third has a stronger claim to such assistance than the first two, based merely on the fact that her suffering arises from a severe physical disability. In particular, the third does not appear to have a stronger *dignity-based* claim for PAD than the others. She finds profound indignity in her physical dependence; the mayor finds it in her mortifying conduct and public exposure; and the entrepreneur finds it in her sons' humiliating treatment. Intuitively, there is no deeper indignity in her severe physical disability than in the others' private humiliation and public disgrace.

It might be argued that the mountaineer has a stronger claim to PAD not because her situation is less dignified but, rather, simply because without assistance, she, unlike the other two, will not be able to secure a dignified death—her disability makes a do-it-yourself suicide nearly impossible. No jurisdiction that permits PAD, however, conditions it on the inability to commit suicide without assistance. Such a requirement would deny claims of PAD to individuals with disabilities that were regarded as highly undignified just so long as they retained the means to end their own misery. The absence of such a "necessity" requirement may reflect the assumption that even the most able-bodied are likely to botch an amateur attempt.[8] Although suicide in not a crime in these jurisdictions, assisting a suicide is a crime, in the absence of a specific exemption.[9]

L. W. Sumner suggests another basis for treating the mountaineer's request differently from those of the others: "Assisted death is a form of medical treatment, and, as such, should be reserved for the relief of suffering due to a medical condition."[10] It is not clear, however, why PAD should be regarded as a medical treatment; why, even if it is a medical treatment, it should be reserved for suffering due to medical conditions; and why the dignity-based suffering of severely disabled people should be regarded as "due to" their medical conditions. Concerning the first, there is a great deal of debate about whether "medical treatment" includes only health-protecting or -restoring interventions or whether it extends to the exercise of medical skill for other purposes, from abortion to execution. Even if it extends to alleviating suffering, it is not clear why the suffering must arise from a medical condition, as long as medical measures are effective in alleviating it. Finally, it is not clear why suffering such as the mountaineer's should be attributed to the physical disability, when it is neither a symptom nor a biological effect of that disability or of the underlying disease process but, rather, a response to that disability – a response that is mediated by a variety of psychological and social factors, notably the individual's willingness and ability to find other sources of meaning and satisfaction in life and the society's willingness and ability to provide them.

A related reason for singling out medical conditions and physical disabilities as causes of unbearable suffering is epistemic: It is far easier for the physicians who make the eligibility determination to ascertain disease or disability than other causes. But this reflects a confusion about what

---

[8] Recall Dorothy Parker's cautionary verse: "Razors pain you; Rivers are damp; Acids stain you; And drugs cause cramp; Guns aren't lawful; Nooses give; Gas smells awful; You might as well live" (*Resumé*).

[9] I thank Adam Cureton for suggesting that I address this argument.

[10] Leonard Wayne Sumner, *Assisted Death: A Study in Ethics and Law* (New York: Oxford University Press, 2011).

must be ascertained. The issue is rarely whether the claimant actually has a disease or physical disability but, rather, whether that condition has caused unbearable and irremediable suffering or whether it is sufficiently undignified to warrant PAD regardless of the magnitude of suffering. Except in cases in which such suffering is attributable to, or constituted by, physical pain (and not necessarily in those cases, either), a physician has no special expertise in judging how much an individual is suffering or in tracing her suffering to a particular source—let alone in assessing the depth of her indignity. In fact, physicians have a well-documented tendency to rate the quality of life of people with physical disabilities far lower than it is rated by those individuals and their families[11]—a tendency that casts doubt on physicians' judgments about the magnitude and source of the suffering or indignity arising from physical disability, even in cases in which individual seek physician assistance to end their lives.

Indeed, there is one respect in which PAD would be *more* problematic for the mountaineer than the other two. Society arguably has greater responsibility for her indignity than it does for the indignity of the entrepreneur or mayor. It could not have prevented the entrepreneur's foolish division of her assets or the mayor's reckless escapade. And although small-town puritanism and sanctimony doubtless contributed to the ex-mayor's humiliation, the reaction to her offense was based at least in part on widely accepted moral values and legal norms. In contrast, the mountaineer's society may bear considerable responsibility for her misery. It may have contributed to her unwarranted sense of shame. It may have perpetuated the pernicious view that the need for assistance in daily activities such as toileting is profoundly demeaning—for example, by the poor compensation and low status of the individuals who provide such assistance, or by the abysmal quality of many of the institutions that provide it. And the enforcement of the laws mandating the inclusion of people with disabilities has been woefully inadequate.

This is not to claim that in a society that treats physically disability justly and respectfully, no one who became disabled would seek to end her life. It is merely to say that such decisions would be far less likely, and that the role of injustice and disrespect in making them more likely should give us the same discomfort about PAD in the third case that we feel in the other two.

The role of social attitudes and practices in creating the indignity experienced by people with severe physical disabilities is well illustrated by

---

[11] See references in Note 7.

the case of *Elizabeth Bouvia v. Superior Court*.[12] In the factual background to the case, the court described both the physical dependence of Elizabeth Bouvia and her family's response to her needs:

> Except for a few fingers of one hand and some slight head and facial movements, she is immobile. She is physically helpless and wholly unable to care for herself. She is totally dependent upon others for all of her needs. These include feeding, washing, cleaning, toileting, turning, and helping her with elimination and other bodily functions. She cannot stand or sit upright in bed or in a wheelchair. She lies flat in bed and must do so the rest of her life. She suffers also from degenerative and severely crippling arthritis. She is in continual pain. Another tube permanently attached to her chest automatically injects her with periodic doses of morphine which relieves some, but not all of her physical pain and discomfort.
>
> She is intelligent, very mentally competent. She earned a college degree. She was married but her husband has left her. She suffered a miscarriage. She lived with her parents until her father told her that they could no longer care for her. She has stayed intermittently with friends and at public facilities. A search for a permanent place to live where she might receive the constant care which she needs has been unsuccessful. She is without financial means to support herself and, therefore, must accept public assistance for medical and other care.[13]

And yet in upholding Bouvia's decision to have her life support withdrawn, the court utterly ignored the role that her family's abandonment and the lack of social support may have played in her predicament:

> Petitioner would have to be fed, cleaned, turned, bedded, toileted by others for 15 to 20 years! Although alert, bright, sensitive, perhaps even brave and feisty, she must lie immobile, unable to exist except through physical acts of others. Her mind and spirit may be free to take great flights but she herself is imprisoned and must lie physically helpless subject to the ignominy, embarrassment, humiliation and dehumanizing aspects created by her helplessness. We do not believe it is the policy of this state that all and every life must be preserved against the will of the sufferer. It is incongruous, if not monstrous, for medical practitioners to assert their right to preserve a life that someone else must live, or, more accurately, endure, for "15 to

---

[12] *Bouvia v. The Superior Court of Los Angeles County* 179 Cal.App.3d 1127–1147 (1986).
[13] *Bouvia v. Superior Court*, 1136.

20 years." We cannot conceive it to be the policy of this state to inflict such an ordeal upon anyone.[14]

It would be difficult to find a more brutal expression of the attitudes the mountaineer has internalized. This passage does less to justify her or Bouvia's suicide than to indict society for the propagation of attitudes that make suicide an appealing option. If society can be regarded as complicit in this way in the mountaineer's perceived indignity, her society has questionable standing to assist in her suicide as a way to escape or mitigate that indignity.[15] Society faces no such moral constraint in the case of the entrepreneur, and it faces less of a constraint, if any, in the case of the mayor. The prevailing judgment of adults who engage in sex with underage partners may be overly harsh and insufficiently nuanced, but it is not invidious.[16]

How Do the Three Cases Fare under Plausible Accounts of Dignity?

Thus far, I used "dignity" and "indignity" in a colloquial or intuitive sense. I have suggested that the indignity felt in cases of physical disability need not be, and often is not, qualitatively greater than that in cases of private or public humiliation and that the case for such assistance may actually be weaker in the former case because of society's greater responsibility for the indignity. But I still need to consider whether there is a plausible and morally weighty sense of dignity in which the mountaineer, but not the mayor or entrepreneur, has a dignity-based claim to PAD. I argue that there is not.

I begin by acknowledging that "dignity" is used in a variety of senses by laypeople and moral philosophers—senses that cannot be assumed to

---

[14] *Bouvia v. Superior Court*, 1143–1144.

[15] Such complicity imposes only limited constraints. Even if it weighs against PAD, it should not override a patient's right to the withdrawal of life-sustaining treatment.

[16] Having won her right to die, Bouvia chose not to act on it. Although she remained ambivalent about life, it became less of an ordeal as her pain management improved and she was enabled to move to a more congenial environment more than a decade after the decision. According to Novella (http://novella.mhhe.com/sites/dl/free/0078038456/1037408/Pen38456_Ch02.pdf), "In 1997, a new pro bono attorney . . . got her disability payments put into a trust fund that allowed her to live in her own apartment with 24-hour-a-day, in-home assistants. Even though this cost far less than her hospital room, it took a decade to accomplish." The moral of her story, as drawn by disability advocates, is that assisted suicide should never be considered as an option in nonterminal cases until the social impediments to a decent life have been addressed.

share a core feature. Such a feature would have to be possessed by both the Kantian notion of dignity invoked to oppose or restrict assisted suicide and the popular notion invoked to demand it as a right. But at the same time, a pluralistic account of "dignity" should be able to suggest why that term is used in such diverse and opposing ways. Moreover, it should be able to explain why an affront to dignity in any familiar sense is a morally serious matter. This would not be the case, for example, if there was no difference, or only one of slight degree, between an indignity and an embarrassment.

Clearly, all three individuals described in the previous section still possess dignity in Kant's own sense; indeed, nothing they could do or suffer could threaten it as long as it left them with the capacity for rational agency. Dignity in that sense, far from justifying assisted suicide, has been invoked to oppose or restrict it. It is the ultimate value *in* the life of a rational agent, not the value of life *for* that agent. The individual has no more, or little more, moral authority to destroy that value than anyone else. Suicide is justified, if at all, only to prevent the loss of that value—for example, to end overwhelming pain, preempt severe dementia, or, arguably, save a greater number of lives.

There are, however, less austere but morally significant senses in which all of them could claim to have lost their dignity. I consider three recent approaches to understanding human dignity—in terms of a coherent or meaningful life narrative; in terms of personal, social, and human standards; and in terms of basic human functioning. Although none of these approaches are fully satisfactory, each captures some of the intuitive moral force of the ordinary notion of dignity. I argue, however, that none provide a basis for treating physical disability differently than other sources of perceived indignity. None support a presumption that severe physical disability is undignified in a way that betrayal, humiliation, and shame are not.

These three approaches to dignity overlap. A life narrative is typically informed by values or standards that the individual attempts to live by and may fail to live up to, and some but not all standards presuppose a minimum level of functioning. But each of the three approaches has a distinct emphasis, which I hope will become clear as I apply them to the three previously discussed cases and to requests for PAD more broadly. The narrative approach evaluates a life over time rather than any particular point in time; it requires both a retrospective and a prospective view. The standards approach focuses on discrete episodes, events, or actions, and it is primarily, although not exclusively, retrospective. The basic-function approach is primarily prospective, examining the individual's present and future capacity to exercise the functions deemed critical to her humanity.

I devote most of the discussion to narrative approaches because they have been the most widely discussed in the context of assisted suicide.

Narrative Dignity

The best known narrative account derives from Ronald Dworkin's controversial discussion of assisted suicide in *Life's Dominion*.[17] Dworkin introduces and defends the notion of an individual's "critical interests" in living a certain kind of life, which may conflict with her merely "experiential interests" in achieving a favorable ratio of pleasure to pain, or reward to frustration.

If the individual loses her capacity to decide for herself, those who make decisions for her should give priority to her critical over her experiential interests when they conflict.

For Dworkin, an individual's critical interests concern the kind of life she has come to believe is "the right one" for her. The idea of integrity is central to understanding these interests:

> The idea that the value of a life lies in part *in* its integrity, so that its having already been established as one kind of life argues, though of course far from conclusively, that it should go on being that kind of life.[18]

Dworkin regards an individual's death as important in two ways to the kind of life she leads or has led. First, "death is the far boundary of life, and every part of our life, including the very last, is important." Second, "death is special, a peculiarly significant event in the narrative of our lives, like the final scene of a play, with everything about it intensified, under a special spotlight."[19] It is in this second way that death is especially important to the individual's critical interests. Dworkin suggests, for example, that those interests are often disserved by the perpetuation of an individual's life when she has lost the capacity for consciousness. Describing the condition of Sonny von Bulow, he states,

> [She] still lies wholly unconscious in a hospital room in Manhattan; every day she is turned and groomed by people willing and paid to do it. She will never respond in any way to that care. It would not have been odd for her to

---

[17] Ronald M. Dworkin, *Life's Dominion: An Argument about Abortion, Euthanasia, and Individual Freedom* (New York: Knopf, 1993).

[18] Dworkin, *Life's Dominion*, 206.

[19] Dworkin, *Life's Dominion*, 209.

think, before she fell into her coma, that this kind of pointless solicitude was insulting, itself an affront to her dignity.[20]

Perhaps some would find such solicitude deeply caring and respectful; Dworkin's point is that it would be inconsistent with the kind of life many other people have chosen for themselves, compromising the integrity of their lives by extending them.

The rigidity of Dworkin's idea of integrity becomes apparent when he considers losses and misfortunes that leave the individual fully conscious, capable of reassessing and revising the values that informed her narrative in light of changed circumstances. Thus, speaking of "athletes, and others whose physical activity was at the center of their self-conception," Dworkin proclaims,

> For such people, a life without the power of motion is unacceptable, not for reasons explicable in experiential terms, but because it is stunningly inadequate to the conception of self around which their lives have so far been constructed. Adding decades of immobility to a life formerly organized around action will for them leave a narrative wreck, with no structure or sense, a life worse than one that ends when its activity ends.[21]

Although he purports to be merely describing the view of "such people," Dworkin appears to find that view eminently reasonable, if not compelling. His tacit endorsement strikes me as a misguided counsel of despair, less hysterical but no more balanced than the opinion of the *Bouvia* court.

Dworkin's stress on the integrity of an individual's unaltered narrative appears to preclude substantial changes in response to critical reflection or adaptation, including the endorsement of changes in values and goals arising from chance disruptions of the original narrative. Dworkin states that "for some," the coherence of a life requires "that it display a steady, self-sustaining commitment to a vision of character or achievement that the life as a whole, seen as an integral creative narrative, illustrates and expresses."[22] Despite the qualification, Dworkin writes as if this "steady, self-sustaining commitment" was important, if not essential, to the integrity of a life.

---

[20] Dworkin, *Life's Dominion*, 210.
[21] Dworkin, *Life's Dominion*, 210–211.
[22] Dworkin, *Life's Dominion*, 205.

Others disagree. Jyl Gentzler, whose own account I discuss later, observes that

> our lives are not entirely subject to our control: We can unexpectedly find ourselves pregnant, we can acquire a chronic illness or disability, a person with whom we planned to spend our life can disappear from our life, we can lose our job, we can lose our home, we can grow old. Such changes in our life situation might be incompatible with our sense of what is valuable; and the life we are forced to lead might be contrary to our present character. As such, they would threaten what Dworkin defines as the "integrity," and hence dignity, of a life. But . . . many people who experience such change in their lives speak of it as initially unwelcome, but ultimately life-enhancing turn of events. To respond effectively to radical change requires courage and spirit, but to muster such traits, it seems to me, enhances rather than threatens one's dignity as a human being.[23]

An insistence on either persevering or dying when one's life narrative confronts such recalcitrant circumstances strikes me as evidence of rigidity, not integrity. Dworkin's emphasis on staying the course is suggested by his declaration that "we think that someone who acts out of character, either for gain or to avoid trouble, has insufficient respect for himself."[24] Much of the adaptation Gentzler describes could be uncharitably characterized as "acting out of character . . . to avoid trouble." Although Dworkin does not say as much, he also gives no indication of recognizing that narrative redirection can be a paradigmatic exercise of self-authorship.

For example, consider the most famous narrative redirection in the Western canon, Saul's conversion on the road to Damascus. Saul was a committed persecutor of Christians; he was heading from Jerusalem to Damascus to arrest any he could find there. On the road, Jesus suddenly appeared to him to ask why he persecuted His followers. Blinded for three days, he was approached in Damascus by Ananias, one of the men he would have arrested:

> Placing his hands on Saul, he said, "Brother Saul, the Lord—Jesus, who appeared to you on the road as you were coming here—has sent me so that you may see again and be filled with the Holy Spirit." Immediately,

---

[23] Jyl Gentzler, "What Is a Death with Dignity?", *Journal of Medicine and Philosophy* 28, no. 4 (2003): 461–487.

[24] Dworkin, *Life's Dominion*, 205.

something like scales fell from Saul's eyes, and he could see again. He got up and was baptized.[25]

Saul changed his name to Paul and went on the become Jesus' apostle to the Gentiles. Dworkin, it seems, would have to find in his conversion a profound loss of integrity. It was, after all, a repudiation of all he had stood and worked for, utterly at odds with the "conception of self around which [his life had] so far been constructed." Clearly, this is not the way the author of Acts regarded Saul's conversion; it was, rather, a critical chapter in the narrative of Paul's life.

The limitations of Dworkin's account become even more apparent if we take seriously his notion of a life narrative as a kind of artistic creation. As he states, "We can, and do, treat leading a life as itself a kind of creative activity, which we have at least as much reason to honor as artistic creation."[26] Like Gentzler, I think that we have particular reason to honor the "artistic creation" of an individual who radically revises her life narrative in the face of circumstances that disrupt it—even when those changes run contrary to her previous character and commitments. Autobiographies that display such adaptability and resourcefulness are at least as admirable, and generally far more interesting, than narratives that run a straight course.[27]

A more nuanced narrative approach is suggested by Thomas Hill in his modified Kantian account of assisted suicide.[28] Hill considers a Consumer perspective on life, akin to Dworkin's experiential view. But he introduces two other perspectives. On the opposite extreme of the Consumer is the Obituarist, who looks at a life "as one might from life's end, preparing to summarize its salient features for the world." Any particular action or event in a life is "measured by its contribution to the whole biography." From this perspective, the decision about whether to end or extend an

---

[25] Acts 9:17–18, *Holy Bible, New International Version* (Grand Rapids, Mich.: Zondervan, 1984).

[26] Dworkin, *Life's Dominion*, 84.

[27] The fidelity to past values and commitments that Dworkin demands of the author unreasonably constrains her present and future choices. If we take Dworkin's claim of life as an artistic creation seriously, we should recognize that an artist's work hardly loses authenticity or integrity if she alters her original vision or plan while the work is still in progress. Sometimes, the changes she makes will be in response to unexpected developments in her life. Indeed, many artists have been driven or inspired by their adversities to greater creative achievement; the obvious example is Beethoven's deafness. Moreover, some acclaimed artistic works have more than one version or ending. We may regard one version or ending as the most unified, original, or brilliant, or regard different versions or endings as incommensurable. But by itself, it does not matter whether one was the original or whether one was responsive to traumatic events in the artist's life.

[28] Thomas E. Hill, "Self-Regarding Suicide: A Modified Kantian View," *Suicide and Life-Threatening Behavior* 13, no. 4 (1983): 254–275.

individual's life depends on whether her continued existence is "a necessary condition for the unfolding of a life of a certain sort."[29] This sounds somewhat like Dworkin's narrative view, in which such a decision should be made on the basis of the individual's critical interest in preserving the integrity of her life. Furthermore, like Dworkin's narrator, the obituarist must work with a constrained narrative—in Dworkin's case, constrained by the narrator's basic values and commitments, and in the obituarist's case, constrained by the fact that the life is viewed as if it is at its end.

Hill, however, offers a third perspective, that of the Author, which is more congenial to adaptation and revision. He states, "As I imagine a working novelist might, this looks both forwards and backwards, wondering what it would be to experience each stretch of life but ever mindful of how it fits into a meaningful whole."[30] What qualifies as a meaningful life is not fixed by the life the individual has previously lead:

> The author, in part, writes the criteria of evaluation as well as the story line. The value of the life as author, when the life is one's own, is not seen as entirely derivative from the final content of the story, once finished. . . . Rather, living as the author, making the crucial choices, deciding what to count as meaningful and what trivial, these are valued for their own sakes."[31]

It is up to the author to determine if a disruption of her prior narrative, whether wrought by others, herself, or circumstances, is important or trivial. She is not constrained by that narrative to view its disruption as catastrophic and irremediable.

In contrast to Dworkin, then, Hill emphasizes the openness of the narrative and the author's prerogative to maintain or change course: "The value in living is not entirely determined by the content of the life one makes; rather, that life acquires value in part because it is the expression of one's choices as an author."[32] From this perspective, the fidelity that Dworkin requires to a past narrative or self-conception serves only to restrict the agent's autonomy.

From Hill's Author perspective, the athlete Dworkin describes might be seen as suffering from writer's block more than quadriplegia. She did

---

[29] Hill, "Self-Regarding Suicide," 98.
[30] Hill, "Self-Regarding Suicide," 99.
[31] Hill, "Self-Regarding Suicide," 99.
[32] Hill, "Self-Regarding Suicide," 99.

not succeed in her attempt to script a satisfactory change in her life narrative; others, similarly situated, might have succeeded. Much the same could be said about the mountaineer, mayor, and entrepreneur. All three suffered from insufficient creativity or resilience as much as from their reversal of fortune; all three of their stories could have had more satisfactory, even uplifting, endings. Those endings, like Saul's conversion, would have been a response to narrative disruptions beyond their control. But like Saul's conversion, those endings would have enhanced, not compromised, the integrity of their authors' lives. I do not want to suggest that they are blameworthy for this failure, let alone that they should be denied PAD because they failed to turn a sow's ear into a silk purse. The lack of creativity or resilience may be as much beyond their control as the events that disrupted their original narratives. My point is that the ultimate failure in each case is one they all share—one that has little or nothing to do with their specific misfortunes, particularly the mountaineer's physical disability.

Personal, Social, and Human Dignity

Suzy Killmister develops a conception of "dignity" in terms of personal, social, and human standards. She attempts to explain how dignity, as commonly understood, can be universal—owed to all human beings—at the same time it is vulnerable and variably achieved, affected by others' actions, by circumstances, and by the agent's own conduct.[33] She analyzes dignity in terms of the imposition of, and adherence to, normative standards: personal standards imposed by the individual on herself; social standards imposed by the community; and human standards, applicable to all individuals recognized as members of the human community. Human standards account for the universality of dignity, although in a more contingent way than rationality does for Kant, because the boundaries of the human community, and the terms of membership, are themselves mutable social constructions. Personal and social standards account for the vulnerability of dignity and its variable achievement: Human agency and circumstances can cause an individual to fall short of the standards she or her community recognizes.

The contingency of personal, social, and even human standards accounts for the undeniable fact that individuals and societies vary widely in what they regard as undignified, and for whom. But recognizing this contingency

---

[33] Suzy Killmister, "Dignity: Personal, Social, Human," *Philosophical Studies* (2016), available online at http://link.springer.com/article/10.1007/s11098-016-0788-y.

does not preclude two kinds of moral criticism. First, we can criticize both personal and social standards as reflecting morally objectionable views about race, class, sex, sexual orientation, and so on, and, as such, incompatible with human standards of dignity. At the same time, we can criticize conduct that causes an individual to fall below social standards, however objectionable. We may, for example, reject a social standard that requires class- and sex-specific dress and that regards it as undignified for individuals to appear in public otherwise attired. But we may also criticize conduct for causing indignity under that objectionable standard. Given that standard of dress, it is an indignity to be forced to dress in nonconforming attire; for example, it is an indignity to force a man to wear women's clothing even though it is also wrong to establish or enforce such a sex-specific dress code. Killmister's account thus allows us to recognize that betrayed, ostracized, and severely disabled individuals do suffer indignities, but at the same time it allows us to criticize the standards under which they do.

For Killmister, the entrepreneur, mayor, and mountaineer have all suffered a loss of dignity. All three fall short of their personal standards: the entrepreneur because of her rash decision and her sons' betrayal; the mayor because of her impulsive act, cruel exposure, and unforgiving community; and the mountaineer simply because of her loss of function. The entrepreneur and the mayor have clearly suffered a loss of social dignity as well; the mountaineer less obviously so. Although she no longer enjoys the renown and admiration she once had, her family, friends, and fans may well be more accepting than she is of her loss of function and need for assistance. Nevertheless, general social standards remain deeply ableist, and many other people doubtless view her situation as undignified. She is likely to be the recipient of pity from acquaintances and furtive stares from strangers—responses that lower her social status and reinforce her self-contempt. All three individuals, of course, are still recognized as members of the human community and accorded the "thin" respect that comes with that recognition.

Dignity as Basic Human Functioning

Gentzler's Aristotelian account of human dignity is based on the functions and capacities that are regarded as conferring or defining humanity:

> All human beings will need to develop their capabilities for effective information-gathering, problem-solving, value-judgment, social interaction, loving intimacy, and control of fear and desire. . . . On Aristotle's view,

the potential for such cognitive and emotional capabilities is part of what makes one human. . . . The exercise of these capabilities is not only instrumental to the satisfaction of basic needs but, in addition, is itself constitutive of a good human life, or *eudemonia*.[34]

Gentzler explains the relationship of these activities to dignity in terms of the virtues realized through these capabilities:

> Although Aristotle does not speak of a life with dignity *per se*, I would suggest that when we speak of a life with dignity, we have in mind a life in which one engages in activities that either develop or exercise the human virtues.[35]

These Aristotelian capabilities, and the resulting virtues, are broadly defined, so that the loss of physical functions need not have an adverse impact on dignity:

> On an Aristotelian view, physical disability does not itself detract from the dignity of a life, but in some social circumstances, it can make it more difficult to exercise one's virtues of thought and character. A society that is concerned with the dignity of human lives will consider the physical needs that must be met if all persons at all stages of their lives are to live their lives with dignity, rather than offer them a right to terminate their existence when past social choices make it impossible for them to exercise their virtues of thought and character.[36]

Gentzler's account, like those of Hill and Killmister, invites us to see the mountaineer's indignity as self-imposed, not by her physical disability but, rather, by her deficit of imagination or resilience. For Gentzler, if anything made the mountaineer undignified, it would not be her physical disability but, rather, her deficient exercise the appropriate virtues in response to it— her inability to display, in the face of frustration and loss, the same high level of courage and perseverance than she previously exercised in the face of formidable physical challenges and dangers. If she had, perhaps she eventually would have found satisfaction in some alternative to the career she lost to her disease. While the application of Gentzler's

---

[34] Gentzler, "Death with Dignity," 476–477.
[35] Gentzler, "Death with Dignity," 477.
[36] Gentzler, "Death with Dignity," 479.

account to the entrepreneur and the mayor may be less clear, they too suffer from a failure or inability to adapt the virtues they had possessed to their new, more difficult, circumstances. We can imagine, for example, the entrepreneur cunningly undermining her sons' financial control, or the mayor redeeming herself through appropriate community service. In all three cases, society could have provided more tangible and intangible resources for them to do so, although, as I suggested, its failure to do so may be more egregious in the case of the mountaineer.

Conclusion

There may be philosophical accounts of human dignity that treat severe physical disability as itself an indignity. But I hope I have shown that such a treatment of disability is suspect and should count against any such account. I have made, and perhaps belabored, the point that severe physical disabilities are just some of the many conditions that can, but need not, contribute to a sense of indignity so profound as to make suicide a reasonable option. A myriad of losses and misfortunes can damage or destroy that which we most value in ourselves, turning us into the kinds of people we would have previously disdained or pitied. There is nothing special about physical disability in this respect, except that the loss of physical function and the accompanying need for physical assistance are especially stigmatized types of misfortune. To single out severe physical disability as a factor that supports a claim for PAD is to reinforce that stigma. This hardly means that individuals cannot adduce their physical disabilities in making a case for PAD by establishing profound indignity or unbearable suffering. My point is merely that those disabilities should have no greater weight, in general or as a category, than other losses that prompt individuals to seek physician assistance in ending their lives.[37]

---

[37] Disclaimer: The views expressed in this chapter are solely the author's. They do not represent the position or policy of the National Institutes of Health, US Public Health Service, or the Department of Health and Human Services.

CHAPTER 7 | Dementia, Dignity, and
Physician-Assisted Death

REBECCA DRESSER

MEDICAL AND PUBLIC health advances have extended the human life-
span, with immense benefit to individuals, families, and societies. But
the advances have also had a negative consequence: More people are living long enough to become affected by Alzheimer's disease and other
age-related dementias. Today, many people are terrified that they might
develop dementia. Indeed, polls in the United States show that dementia
could soon displace cancer as the disease people dread most.[1]

Fear of dementia has provoked a debate about whether physician-
assisted death (PAD), a term encompassing physician-assisted suicide and
voluntary active euthanasia, should be available to people at risk of or
diagnosed with dementia. So far, lawmakers in most countries have failed
to authorize PAD for dementia. There are a few exceptions, however. The
Netherlands and Belgium have legalized PAD for some individuals preferring death over life with dementia.[2]

People in favor of allowing PAD for dementia offer several justifications
for their position. As in the general campaign to legalize PAD, preservation
of dignity is a central theme. Yet dignity and assisted death have a complicated relationship with regard to potential or actual dementia patients.

---

[1] See Mario Garrett, "Fear of Dementia," *iAge Blog*, May 11, 2013. Retrieved July 1, 2016, from
https://www.psychologytoday.com/blog/iage/201305/fear-dementia; "Americans Rank Alzheimer's
as Most Feared Disease," November 13, 2012. Retrieved July 1, 2016, from http://www.
helpforalzheimersfamilies.com/alzheimers-dementia-care-services/alzheimers_feared_disease.
[2] Inez D. de Beaufort and Suzanne van der Vathorst, "Dementia and Assisted Suicide and
Euthanasia," *Journal of Neurology* 263, no.7 (2016): 1463–1467; Marike de Boer et al., "Advance
Directives for Euthanasia in Dementia: Do Law-Based Opportunities Lead to More Euthanasia?"
Health Policy 98, no. 2–3 (2010): 256–262.

Dignity may be invoked to justify assisted death for at-risk asymptomatic individuals, as well as for individuals diagnosed with dementia. In this context, requests for PAD rest on an anticipated loss of dignity rather than the contemporaneous loss that motivates most people seeking PAD.

In this chapter, I examine arguments for and against permitting PAD for dementia. I consider the role of dignity concerns in addressing (1) requests for assisted death as a preemptive measure to avoid a possible future with dementia, (2) requests for assisted death by individuals with mild or moderate dementia, and (3) advance directives requesting assisted death when specific manifestations of late-stage dementia appear (e.g., an apparent inability to recognize family and friends). I focus on future-oriented dignity claims and dignity claims by people with reduced intellectual capacities.

Changing Public Conceptions of Death with Dignity

The death with dignity movement began in the 1960s. In the early years, death with dignity advocates campaigned for laws protecting the individual's right to be free of modern medical interventions that could sustain life. Control over the dying process was a major theme of the campaign.

Another early theme was the dehumanizing dimension of artificial life support. For many, the tubes and machines used to maintain life transformed human existence into something strange and disturbing. At that time, dignified death was synonymous with natural death. Death with dignity advocates argued that patients should be permitted to choose a death free of artificial and degrading interference with the natural dying process.

The death with dignity campaign recognized that mental impairments related to illness could deprive patients of the capacity to articulate their end-of-life preferences. Advocates endorsed living wills and other advance medical directives as measures to address this common situation. Through completing a directive, competent individuals could describe their personal conception of dignified death. Family members and clinicians could then forgo interventions that would conflict with the incapacitated patient's formerly stated views. Most ethicists and lawmakers agreed that those at the bedside should strive to respect the individual patient's previously expressed ideas on dignified care at the end of life.[3]

---

[3] Rebecca Dresser, "Autonomy and Its Limits in End-of-Life Law," in *The Oxford Handbook of U.S. Health Law*, ed. I. Glenn Cohen, Allison K. Hoffman, and William M. Sage (New York: Oxford University Press, 2016), 399–420.

These developments addressed many end-of-life concerns but not all of them. Enduring a natural death at times subjected patients to unwanted pain and distress. Waiting for natural death could involve unacceptable suffering—suffering that could interfere with a dignified death. A desire to spare patients this hardship generated support for giving certain patients a means to end their lives before natural death would occur. Advocates taking this position thought that physicians should be allowed to provide the necessary life-ending assistance.

The initial campaign to permit PAD focused on patients facing an inevitable death from natural causes. Terminally ill patients not dependent on life-sustaining interventions could not secure an earlier death through refusing medical care. For some terminally ill patients, death with dignity *required* active medical intervention.

Advocates of PAD argued that competent terminally ill patients should have access to lethal medication so that they could control when they died. At minimum, physicians should be permitted to prescribe medication that patients could take when continued life became intolerable (the practice known as physician-assisted suicide). Some argued that physicians should also be permitted to administer life-ending medication to patients who wanted to die but were physically or emotionally unable to act on their own (the practice known as voluntary euthanasia).

With this debate, dignified death and natural death became two separate ideas, overlapping in some cases but not others. For PAD supporters, individual control over dying was the defining feature of a dignified death. Accordingly, patients should be free to choose an unnatural death through lethal medication if they believed that was necessary to secure a dignified death.

Authorities in different countries responded differently to this development. Although the original death with dignity movement began in the United States, authorities in this country have been slow to accept PAD. The US Supreme Court ruled in 1997 that the US Constitution did not protect the terminally ill person's access to lethal medication. Most of the Supreme Court justices said that the constitutional right to dignified death encompassed a right to refuse life-sustaining treatment, as well as a right to receive necessary pain-relieving measures that might hasten a patient's death. But none of the justices were convinced that access to PAD was essential to protecting this right.[4]

---

[4] *Vacco v. Quill,* 521 U.S. 793 (1997).

The Supreme Court ruling left states free to enact laws expanding patients' rights to dignified death, however, and some states have moved in that direction. In those states, statutes and court decisions allow physicians to prescribe lethal medication in narrow circumstances. Eligible patients are competent terminally ill individuals with six months or less to live. In legalizing physician-assisted suicide, officials agreed that for a small group of patients, natural death could be inconsistent with dignified death. But so far, no state has moved to permit any form of PAD for dementia.

Officials in a few countries have taken a more liberal position on PAD. The Netherlands is a leader in this regard. Dutch physicians are legally permitted to supply a wide group of people with life-ending drugs. Assisted death is acceptable in the following circumstances: (1) The patient makes a voluntary and well-considered request, (2) the patient is experiencing unbearable and hopeless suffering, (3) the physician has thoroughly informed the patient about his or her situation and prospects, (4) the physician and patient agree that there is no reasonable alternative to PAD, and (5) at least one consultant physician has examined the patient and provided an opinion on whether the previous criteria have been met. One of the law's provisions allows a patient's advance directive request for PAD to substitute for a contemporaneous request for assisted death.[5]

Dutch law permits both physician-assisted suicide and voluntary active euthanasia. The law requires physicians to exercise "due care" in determining which individuals qualify for assisted dying. Cases are reviewed by a committee to ensure that physicians apply the legal criteria.[6] As I describe later, Dutch law has been interpreted to allow PAD for dementia in limited circumstances.

Physician-assisted death for people with dementia presents distinct controversies in the effort to promote death with dignity. Addressing these controversies requires a close examination of the meaning of human dignity and its potential relevance to end-of-life decisions. Although dignity analysis fails to supply clear answers to the controversies, it highlights and clarifies the moral issues at stake.

---

[5] Marike E. de Boer et al., "Advance Directives in Dementia: Issues of Validity and Effectiveness," *International Psychogeriatrics* 22, no. 2 (2010): 201–208.
[6] Cees M. P. M. Hertogh, "The Role of Advance Euthanasia Directives as an Aid to Communication and Shared Decision-Making in Dementia," *Journal of Medical Ethics* 35, no. 2 (2009): 100–103.

Dignity in Bioethics

Bioethics analysis often cites the importance of human dignity, yet writers disagree on the concept's meaning and significance. Some state that human dignity is equivalent to more foundational values, such as individual autonomy and respect for persons. From this perspective, the concept of human dignity adds nothing substantive to bioethics debates.[7]

Yet efforts to dismiss the concept of dignity have been unsuccessful. Dignity may have its critics, but it has many defenders as well. Defenders contend that a bioethics without dignity would be both conceptually anemic and morally inadequate.[8]

Scholars defending the role of dignity in bioethics often focus on end-of-life care. Much of this work refers to two dimensions of dignity. One dimension is subjective, reflecting the individual person's idea of dignified death. The other dimension is general, applicable to all human beings.

Daryl Pullman's 2004 article, "Death, Dignity, and Moral Nonsense," is a useful articulation of this approach.[9] Pullman believes that the concept of dignity is crucial to moral decision-making, as well as to policy determinations about appropriate end-of-life options. He also believes that two different conceptions of dignity are relevant to moral and policy analysis. "Personal dignity" is closely related to individual control and autonomy over end-of-life decisions. Honoring dignity in this sense requires giving great weight to the preferences of individuals making life-and-death choices.

But Pullman argues that a second conception of dignity is also essential in determining permissible end-of-life practices. What Pullman calls "basic dignity" demands that "we recognize humans as possessors of intrinsic and inalienable moral worth."[10] Basic dignity applies equally to all humans, no matter what their capacities and circumstances. Dignity in this sense is universal and cannot be taken away from anyone. And basic dignity sets limits on expressions of personal dignity. On this analysis,

---

[7] Ruth Macklin, "Dignity Is a Useless Concept," *BMJ* 327, no. 7429 (2003): 1419–1420; Alasdair Cochrane, "Undignified Bioethics," *Bioethics* 24, no. 5 (2010): 234–241.
[8] For example, Inmaculada de Melo-Martin, "An Undignified Bioethics: There Is No Method in This Madness," *Bioethics* 26, no. 4 (2012): 224–230; Suzy Killmister, "Dignity: Not Such a Useless Concept," *Journal of Medical Ethics* 36, no. 3 (2010): 160–164; Rebecca Dresser, "Dignity Can Be a Useful Concept in Bioethics," in *Bioethics, Public Moral Argument, and Social Responsibility*, ed. Nancy M. P. King and Michael J. Hyde (New York: Routledge, 2012), 45–54.
[9] Daryl Pullman, "Death, Dignity, and Moral Nonsense," *Journal of Palliative Care* 20, no. 3 (2004): 171–178.
[10] Pullman, "Death, Dignity, and Moral Nonsense," 172.

we are not required to honor end-of-life choices that conflict with basic dignity.

For Pullman, basic dignity underlies a moral mandate to "accept that all human beings have implicit moral worth and are, thus, worthy of moral consideration."[11] Basic dignity supplies moral grounds for condemning certain behavior, such as consensual human cannibalism. But Pullman thinks basic dignity might accommodate at least some PAD applications. He contends that basic dignity gives the moral community a degree of leeway to determine when PAD is acceptable. As he sees it, society's conception of basic dignity "is to some extent shaped and altered by the various expressions of personal dignity which are permitted and tolerated over time."[12] Different visions of basic dignity are being offered in current debates over PAD for dementia; the vision that prevails will influence "the way we think about ourselves as moral creatures, both now and in the future."[13]

Does basic dignity permit PAD for individuals who regard dementia as a threat to personal dignity? This question underlies much of the debate over PAD and dementia. People who view dementia as such a threat may prefer an early death over life with dementia. But scholars and policymakers disagree on whether permitting PAD for these individuals would be acceptable in light of society's obligation to protect the basic dignity of dementia patients.

Dementia and Physician-Assisted Death: Dignity-Based Arguments

Requests for immediate PAD to avoid dementia are made by (1) asymptomatic individuals who learn they are at higher than average risk of developing dementia and (2) individuals diagnosed with early dementia. Dementia can also be the basis of a request for future PAD. Through completing an advance euthanasia directive (AED), individuals express a wish to receive life-ending medication when progressive dementia causes a loss of dignity. Such directives could appeal to any person who believes that dementia will at some point eliminate the possibility of dignified life.

---

[11] Pullman, "Death, Dignity, and Moral Nonsense," 175.

[12] Pullman, "Death, Dignity, and Moral Nonsense," 176.

[13] Pullman, "Death, Dignity, and Moral Nonsense," 177.

The Indignities of Dementia

It is not unusual for people to associate dementia with an undignified existence. The legal philosopher Ronald Dworkin did so openly and graphically, writing that he and approximately half the people he consulted were "repelled by the idea of living demented, totally dependent lives, speaking gibberish, incapable of understanding that there is a world beyond them, let alone of following its course."[14]

Other writers agree that the prospect of living with dementia can be unbearable. People suffer because they know "what the disease will do to one's personality and life."[15] They dread the "loss of self, a condition of such indignity in the minds of some that life would not be worth living."[16]

Dignity and related concepts, such as autonomy and control, supply the moral basis for permitting PAD to avoid dementia. Choosing PAD for dementia is viewed as an essential part of the individual's right to make important personal and medical decisions.[17] According to Dworkin and his allies, competent individuals have morally important interests in living the final stages of life in a manner consistent with the values that shaped their earlier lives. People supporting PAD claim that those interests, which Dworkin labels "critical" interests, should be given great weight in determining acceptable end-of-life practices.

Defenders of PAD for dementia say that the competent individual's existing sense of dignity should be respected. As they see it, dementia patients gradually lose their dignity, and patients who have reached an advanced stage have no dignity at all. From this perspective, PAD presents no danger to patients. In the words of one PAD defender, there is "no point at all in continuing my life when I have lost the dignity, the purposes and the emotional commitments that I consider essential to the story of my life and my person."[18]

As noted previously, the Netherlands has made PAD available to certain individuals seeking to counter dementia's threat to their dignity. Dutch law allows physicians to provide lethal medication to some people in the initial

---

[14] Ronald Dworkin, *Life's Dominion: An Argument about Abortion, Euthanasia, and Individual Freedom* (New York: Knopf, 1993), 231.

[15] de Beaufort and van der Vathorst, "Dementia and Assisted Suicide," 2.

[16] Stephen Post, "Physician-Assisted Suicide in Alzheimer's Disease," *Journal of the American Geriatrics Society* 45, no. 5 (1997): 647–651.

[17] Paul Menzel and Bonnie Steinbock, "Advance Directives, Dementia, and Physician-Assisted Death," *Journal of Law, Medicine & Ethics* 41, no. 2 (2013): 484–500.

[18] Inez de Beaufort, "The View from Before," *American Journal of Bioethics* 7, no. 4 (2007): 57–66.

stages of dementia. Dutch law also includes a specific provision permitting physicians to honor advance directives requesting PAD. Thus, Dutch law appears to accept Dworkin's view that the critical interests underlying PAD requests justify assisted death for those who fear dementia's effects.[19]

Doubts about Immediate Physician-Assisted Death for Dementia

Although there is scholarly and legal support for making PAD available to people seeking to avoid the indignities of life with dementia, the support is far from unanimous. Commentators raise many concerns about PAD for dementia, and authorities in most countries remain unpersuaded that the practice should be legalized.

Critics point to several issues that can arise in evaluating dementia-related requests for PAD. Certain features of these requests weaken the case for permitting PAD to protect the dignity of people at risk of or diagnosed with dementia.

In the dementia context, dignity-based requests for assisted death are forward-looking. Individuals seek either an immediate death to avoid what they fear will become an undignified existence or a guarantee that their lives will be ended once they enter that undignified state. The anticipatory nature of their dignity claims gives rise to a number of problems.

Individuals requesting PAD for dementia are acting on a prediction. They believe that the condition condemns them to future indignity. Yet their predictions may be inaccurate. Both requests for immediate PAD and advance directives seeking PAD rely on questionable evidence about dementia's likely impact.

One set of problems arises because presymptomatic testing provides imprecise information about a person's risk of developing dementia. Except in cases involving relatively rare autosomal dominant genetic conditions, preclinical tests are of limited predictive value.[20] Biomarker and other predictive tests for Alzheimer's disease can indicate that a person is at higher than average risk of developing the condition. But not all individuals with above-average risk develop Alzheimer's disease. Some die of other conditions before exhibiting symptoms, and so-called "cognitive reserve" enables others to avoid the impairments associated with Alzheimer's disease. Making immediate PAD available in these circumstances could

---

[19] de Boer et al., "Advance Directives in Dementia."
[20] See Rebecca Dresser, "A Fate Worse Than Death? How Biomarkers for Alzheimer's Disease Could Affect End-of-Life Choices," *Indiana Health Law Review* 12, no. 2 (2015): 651–669.

result in the deaths of many individuals who would never have developed dementia.

The situation is slightly different for individuals who have received a diagnosis of early dementia. People in this group have a higher likelihood of developing the serious memory loss and other deficits that accompany later-stage dementia. But the progression of Alzheimer's disease and other forms of dementia varies widely. If PAD is available to people in the early stages of dementia, many will die long before the point at which they would consider their lives to be undignified.

Other problems with PAD for dementia relate to the general requirements for medical decision-making. According to accepted ethical and legal standards, people making medical decisions should be both competent and informed. Criteria for competency vary, but it is generally agreed that individuals should be capable of understanding the risks and potential benefits of their medical options. Individuals in the early stages of dementia may no longer have that capacity. Empirical studies provide evidence that a considerable number of people with mild dementia are unable to appreciate the possible consequences of their medical choices, give rational reasons for their choices, or demonstrate a good understanding of the information relevant to their choices.[21]

A further question concerns the appropriate competency standard for decisions based on a person's desire to avoid a future state. To make a forward-looking choice for PAD, people must be capable of understanding what it could be like to live as a person with dementia. This kind of decision-making requires people to imagine how they will experience life when their interests and abilities are different from their current ones. This is a more sophisticated kind of thinking than contemporaneous choice requires, and it may be beyond the ability of many people in the early stages of dementia. A study in the United Kingdom found that relatively few subjects with dementia were capable of completing an advance treatment directive.[22]

The evaluation of decision-making capacity is one necessary step in determining the quality of a person's medical choice. Another step is to evaluate the competent person's actual understanding of the important information bearing on that choice. The demand for informed

---

[21] For example, J. H. T. Karlawish et al., "The Ability of Persons with Alzheimer Disease (AD) to Make a Decision about Taking an AD Treatment," *Neurology* 64, no. 9 (2005): 1514–1519.

[22] Seema Fazel, Tony Hope, and Robin Jacoby, "Assessment of Competence to Complete Advance Directives: Validation of a Patient Centred Approach," *BMJ* 318 (1999): 493–497.

decision-making presents challenges to those supporting PAD for dementia, for the facts about one's possible future as a person with dementia are complex.

Negative stereotypes about life with dementia are widespread. Many people are unaware of the good quality of life that patients often experience. Experts point to the declining insight that comes with the condition's progression, as well as dementia patients' tendency to adjust to their changed situations. As geriatric ethicist Cees Hertogh has observed, "people with dementia often come to terms with the consequences of their disease and adapt" to their new circumstances.[23] According to Peter Rabins, a US physician with years of experience working with Alzheimer's patients, people seeking an earlier death over life with dementia are "overestimating the importance of cognition in their lives and underestimating the importance of interpersonal relationships."[24]

People seeking PAD to avoid dementia should have a reasonable understanding of the condition. This includes not only facts about its likelihood and progression but also facts about the subjective experiences of people with dementia. Individuals should understand that dementia will lead them to respond to the world in new ways. Activities and interactions that now appear boring or silly might later be enjoyable. Relationships with spouses and other family members might be better than expected.[25] People cannot be sure how they will fare as dementia patients, but they should understand that people often adapt to an existence that is very different from the one they once valued.

Certainly there is a dark side to having dementia, but the picture is not as dark as many people think. Should immediate PAD be available to protect personal dignity claims that could be misguided, either because the people making those claims might never develop dementia or because they might be content with their quality of life as dementia patients?

Distinct Issues Raised by Advance Euthanasia Directives

Advance directives for PAD present even more challenges than requests for immediate PAD present. People making AEDs must not only meet the customary standards for competent and informed decision-making but

---

[23] Hertogh, "The Role of Advance Euthanasia Directives," 101.
[24] Peter Rabins, "Can Suicide Be a Rational and Ethical Act in Persons with Early or Pre-dementia?" *American Journal of Bioethics* 7, no. 6 (2007): 47–49, 49.
[25] See, for example, N. R. Kleinfield, "Fraying at the Edges," Special Section, *New York Times*, May 1, 2016.

also establish the point at which assisted death should occur. In essence, they must describe the features of what they view as an undignified life with dementia.

People making AEDs for dementia could choose from among a variety of possible activation criteria. An inability to recognize one's family is a particularly terrifying feature of dementia, so it could be a popular choice as the event that should trigger PAD. But to detect this inability, clinicians would have to make subtle judgments about a dementia patient's mental state. Patents unable to specify the names or identities of friends and family members often exhibit behavioral responses suggesting some level of recognition. For example, I have an aunt with dementia who is always delighted to see me. She does not know my name and sometimes refers to me as her cousin. I think she recognizes that I am a relative, but it is impossible to know for sure. I suspect there are many cases like this, in which it is difficult to discern whether a patient can distinguish loved ones from strangers.

To get around a problem such as this, people making AEDs could select different activation criteria, such as the need to move to a nursing home or loss of the ability to walk. Criteria such as these would be easier to apply than criteria that require others to assess a patient's subjective awareness. Yet activation criteria such as these remain morally controversial, for patients in nursing homes and wheelchairs can retain interests in continuing their lives. Would it be acceptable to allow PAD for such patients?

This question brings us to the most significant moral challenge AEDs present: determining the authority that competent individuals should have over their future lives as dementia patients.[26] Patients who have lost the capacity to make medical decisions remain able to enjoy and appreciate life. As Dworkin recognized, they retain experiential interests that can give them a stake in continued life. Most people with dementia seem to accept their new situations. Although they often show signs of intermittent distress, much of the time they appear to be content. There are exceptions, but changes in caregiving approaches and care settings can often address patients' apparent unhappiness. And clinicians state they rarely observe clear pain and suffering in later-stage dementia patients.

---

[26] Some of these issues apply as well when people make traditional advance directives refusing treatment if they are incompetent and have dementia. For further discussion, see Rebecca Dresser, "Dworkin on Dementia: Elegant Theory, Questionable Policy," *Hastings Center Report* 27, no. 2 (1995): 34–42.

Are advance requests for PAD sufficient justification for ending the lives of patients who appear unconcerned about the indignities of life with dementia? Such patients' current existence may depart from their once-held conceptions of a dignified life, but they are no longer in touch with those beliefs. In such circumstances, patients' existing experiential interests, together with societal obligations to protect basic human dignity, undermine the case for allowing AEDs for dementia.

Evidence from Dutch Practice

Both the justifications and the concerns I have previously described appear to influence Dutch doctors' willingness to perform PAD to avoid life with dementia. Public records, empirical studies, and case reports supply information about how the law is applied in cases involving dementia.

The Dutch law permitting PAD took effect in 2002. In the early years, few PAD cases involved dementia-based requests. A 2007 article reviewed five known cases in which dementia was the declared reason for PAD. In each case, authorities accepted physicians' findings that the patients were competent and experiencing hopeless and unbearable suffering. Their judgments relied on the assumption that "patients in a very early stage of dementia can still have enough awareness to suffer unbearably from the prospect of increasing mental decline."[27]

But authors of the case review raised several questions about the findings. The reported evidence failed to establish that some of the patients actually had dementia. Some patients also made their PAD requests years after their dementia diagnosis, raising questions about their ability to make capable and informed end-of-life requests.[28]

Despite reservations about the application of PAD in cases such as these, Dutch physicians' willingness to provide immediate PAD for dementia is on the rise. Assisted suicide or euthanasia was granted to forty-nine people with dementia in 2009; by 2013, the number had risen to ninety-seven.

[27] Cees M. P. M. Hertogh et al., "Would We Rather Lose Our Life Than Our Self? Lessons from the Dutch Debate on Euthanasia for Dementia Patients," *American Journal of Bioethics* 7, no. 4 (2007): 48–56, 51.

[28] For articles raising concerns about the quality of Dutch and Belgian physicians' evaluations of requests from people with psychiatric conditions, see Scot Y. H. Kim, Raymond de Vries, and John R. Peteet, "Euthanasia and Assisted Suicide of Patients with Psychiatric Disorders in the Netherlands 2011 to 2014," *JAMA Psychiatry* 73, no. 4 (2016): 362–368; Rachel Aviv, "The Death Treatment," *The New Yorker,* June 22, 2015. Retrieved November 21, 2016, from http://www. newyorker.com/magazine/2015/06/22/the-death-treatment.

Reports show that nearly all of the cases involved people with early dementia who were deemed capable of making their own decisions.[29] Physicians and reviewers apparently believed that the patients were competent and experiencing unbearable suffering that could not be relieved by alternatives to PAD.

Although Dutch physicians are granting more dementia-based requests for PAD, they do not always agree to such requests. Evidence of a mixed picture comes from a study that reviewed reports on 645 Dutch PAD requests from 2012 and 2013. In fifty-six of the cases, individuals cited cognitive decline as the reason for the request. Approximately one-third of those requests were granted, and approximately one-third were rejected. (The remaining requests were withdrawn or the patients died before the PAD decision was made.) Researchers did not have access to material explaining why requests were rejected, but they suspected that patients' lack of decision-making capacity was a common reason.[30]

Moreover, although Dutch physicians are apparently willing to perform immediate PAD for at least some people seeking to avoid further cognitive decline, they are much less inclined to act on AEDs for dementia. As of mid-2016, just one such case had been publicized. The case involved a sixty-four-year-old woman with advanced Alzheimer's disease. After her initial diagnosis, she reportedly told her doctor and family she "was terrified of her illness progressing to the point where she wouldn't recognize them and would have to be admitted to a nursing home."[31] Five years after her diagnosis, she completed an AED, and after that, she continued to insist she wanted to die. Doctors said that she repeatedly expressed this desire in her final months, although by then she did not remember the specifics of her AED. In this case, doctors and the review board concluded that her PAD requests were voluntary and considered.

This case was a stark deviation from usual practice. In surveys and interviews, Dutch physicians have voiced great skepticism about AEDs for dementia. Dutch law allows advance requests to substitute for contemporaneous requests, but the other legal requirements for PAD still apply. Before acting on an advance request, physicians must confirm the patient's unbearable suffering, as well as the absence of any alternative ways to

[29] de Beaufort and van de Vathorst, "Dementia and Assisted Suicide."
[30] Marianne C. Snijdewind et al., "A Study of the First Year of the End-of-Life Clinic for Physician-Assisted Dying in the Netherlands," *JAMA Internal Medicine* 175, no. 10 (2015): 1633–1640.
[31] Tony Sheldon, "Dementia Patient's Suicide Was Lawful, Say Dutch Authorities," *BMJ* 343 (2011): 7510.

reduce it. Many physicians state that patients' loss of communication abilities makes it very difficult to meet these requirements.

In explaining their failure to act on AEDs, Dutch physicians often cite the need for joint decision-making when an AED is activated. In their view, dementia patients who cannot engage in meaningful conversation are not suitable candidates for PAD. As one research group commented, AEDs "were developed for situations in which the patient is no longer able to actively communicate a request for euthanasia, but exactly this lack of in-depth communication seems to be the crucial factor in [Dutch physicians'] non-compliance with [AEDs]."[32]

Delineating Basic Dignity for Dementia Patients

Dignity judgments will undoubtedly play a role in policy decisions about PAD for dementia. Although some people think that personal dignity is the only relevant moral and policy consideration, this view is unlikely to prevail. Permitting PAD for dementia is not simply a matter of respecting individual choice. Authorizing physicians to provide lethal medication to patients signifies that this conduct is consistent with broader social norms and values. Conceptions of basic dignity are bound to affect decisions on whether to allow PAD for dementia.

An example of this thinking comes from philosophers Paul Menzel and Bonnie Steinbock. Although they defend limited PAD for dementia, they also believe that dementia patients are owed dignified treatment. In the following passage, they defend the basic dignity of dementia patients, including those in the late stages of the illness:

> The notion of dignity applicable in dementia . . . has to do with more than present capacities. We respect the person now in part because of what she was— an autonomous, self-constituting, self-conscious narrative self— and because of the narrative identity she still has. But we respect the person also because of the remaining consciousness present in late-stage dementia, and because of her continuing role in a network of relations. The patient with dementia is still someone's husband or wife, someone's mother or father, grandmother or grandfather. Dementia does not banish someone from the human family, nor from their more immediate families.[33]

---

[32] de Boer et al, "Advance Directives for Euthanasia," 261.

[33] Menzel and Steinbock, "Advance Directives, Dementia," 492.

The task ahead is to formulate a defensible response to people seeking PAD to avoid the indignities they associate with dementia. Can such claims be reconciled with the basic dignity protection owed to people with dementia? In the coming years, law and policy will articulate society's response to this question.[34] Public officials are likely to adopt different positions, with some countries agreeing that PAD for dementia is consistent with basic dignity, and others labeling PAD an unacceptable departure from basic dignity obligations.

Moving forward, the debate over PAD for dementia should expressly address three matters. The first involves requests for immediate PAD to avoid future dementia. Decisions based on personal dignity require a reasonable level of understanding about the relevant facts. No country should authorize PAD for dementia without building in meaningful safeguards to prevent life-ending decisions based on confusion, ignorance, or erroneous ideas about the lives of people with dementia.

To prevent misguided decisions, laws permitting PAD for dementia should require rigorous capacity assessment for individuals seeking immediate PAD to avoid the indignities of dementia. Such laws should also require that individuals seeking PAD have a reasonable understanding of the facts about life with dementia. Laws should include mandates to inform people about dementia's progression and the ways that people experience the condition. Such discussions should incorporate insights from people living with dementia and give individuals considering PAD opportunities to spend time with those who actually have the condition.

Second, the debate over AEDs for dementia should directly confront the conflicting values at stake. The competent individual's wish to avoid the indignities of dementia can conflict with the individual's welfare as a dementia patient. Decisions to authorize AEDs for dementia have moral costs—costs that should be openly acknowledged.

Giving effect to personal dignity claims embodied in an AED could have disturbing consequences. A Dutch commentary stated it well:

> Imagine how this would be done in [the] case of an incompetent but still alert and conscious patient with advanced dementia, to whom we cannot explain that in a long forgotten past this was what he wanted to happen to the demented person he has now become.[35]

---

[34] Evan Simpson, "Harms to Dignity, Bioethics, and the Scope of Biolaw," *Journal of Palliative Care* 20, no. 3 (2004): 185–200.

[35] Cees M. P. M. Hertogh et al., "Beyond a Dworkinean View on Autonomy and Advance Directives in Dementia," *American Journal of Bioethics* 7, no. 4 (2007): W4–W6, W5.

To describe this as a straightforward decision to honor the person's advance directive is to adopt "a misleading euphemism for killing a person with dementia."[36]

Attitudes about the value of life with disabilities have evolved in recent decades. Euthanizing dementia patients in the absence of clear threats to their contemporaneous well-being would be a departure from generally accepted views on our obligations to vulnerable people. People who support AEDs for dementia must explain why those obligations should be put aside when they conflict with a PAD request made "in a long forgotten past." Legalization proponents must also address the potential negative effects on clinicians and families of a mandate to end patients' lives based on such past requests.

Third, debates over PAD for dementia should consider dignity and dementia in a broader frame of reference. The disease model of dementia focuses on deficits produced by abnormalities in the brain. But patients' perceptions and behavior are also affected by environmental and social conditions. The difficulties people with dementia encounter are strongly influenced by how others treat them and by the settings in which they live. Changes in these areas could substantially reduce the indignities associated with dementia.

British psychologist Tom Kitwood pioneered the concept of dignity-preserving care for people with dementia.[37] Many have followed his lead in calling for caregivers and others to value what people with dementia can do, such as live in the present and respond with an honesty rarely seen in cognitively "normal" people.[38]

By making an effort to understand the dementia patient's perspective, people can vastly improve the patient's quality of life and sense of dignity.[39] Some communities are creating programs to teach merchants and members of the general public about the best ways to communicate with

---

[36] Hertogh et al., "Beyond a Dworkinean View," W5.

[37] B. Woods, "The Legacy of Professor Tom Kitwood 1937–1998," *Aging & Mental Health* 3, no. 1 (1999): 5–7; Tom Kitwood and Kathleen Bredin, "Towards a Theory of Dementia Care: Personhood and Well-Being," *Ageing & Society* 12, no. 3 (1992): 269–287.

[38] For example, see Steven Sabat, "The Person with Dementia as Understood through Stern's Critical Personalism," in *Beyond Loss: Dementia, Identity, Personhood*, ed. Lars-Christer Hyden, Hilde Lindemann, and Jens Brockmeier (New York: Oxford University Press, 2014), 24–38; Steven Sabat, "Voices of Alzheimer's Disease Sufferers: A Call for Treatment Based on Personhood," *Journal of Clinical Ethics* 9, no. 1 (1998): 35–48. For a description of how the approach works in practice, see Rebecca Mead, "The Sense of an Ending," *The New Yorker*, May 20, 2013, 92–103.

[39] Anne Kari T. Heggestad, Per Nortvedt, and Ashild Slettebo, "'Like a Prison without Bars': Dementia and Experiences of Dignity," *Nursing Ethics* 20, no. 8 (2013): 881–892.

people affected by dementia.[40] Other efforts focus on improving palliative care for advanced dementia patients, for research suggests that symptoms of pain and distress in such patients often go untreated.[41] Better palliative care for people with advanced dementia would reduce their suffering and elevate their dignity.

Responses such as these would also affect how asymptomatic individuals and early stage dementia patients think about dementia and dignity. Efforts to promote patients' well-being could counter "one-sided ideas of elderly people who are scared of dementia."[42] If dementia became a less stigmatizing condition, people might be less worried about a future loss of dignity. They might be less likely to seek preemptive PAD and less likely to make advance directives requesting euthanasia.

Dementia is not purely a medical problem; it is also a cultural problem. In the United States and Europe, dementia and aging signify decline and degradation, fortifying people's worries about their later years. Indeed, the Dutch government has announced it is working on a measure that would make PAD available to healthy older people who would prefer death over the loneliness and dependence they are experiencing.[43]

Decisions to legalize PAD for dementia reinforce individual dread about a future loss of dignity. But there are other ways to respond. The public conversation about PAD and dementia should consider the social factors that influence conceptions of personal dignity. Permitting PAD is not the only way to promote dignity for people at risk of or diagnosed with dementia.

---

[40] See Nuffield Council on Bioethics, "Dementia: Ethical Issues" (2009), available at http://nuffieldbioethics.org/blog/lets-talk-some-more-about-dementia (describing the community's ethical obligation to accept people with dementia and provide services adapted to their needs). See also Sarah Walker-Robinson, *Let's Talk (Some More) about Dementia*, June 17, 2014, available at http://blog.nuffieldbioethics.org/?p=1279.

[41] Hertogh et al., "Would We Rather Lose Our Life."

[42] Hertogh et al., "Would We Rather Lose Our Life," 54.

[43] See Dan Bilefsky and Christopher Schuetze, "Dutch Law Would Allow Assisted Suicide for Healthy Older People," *New York Times*, October 13, 2016. Retrieved October 18, 2016, from http://www.nytimes.com/2016/10/14/world/europe/dutch-law-would-allow-euthanasia-for-healthy-elderly-people.html.

SECTION 4 | Dignity and Autonomy

CHAPTER 8 | Autonomy and the Value of Life as Elements of Human Dignity

SEBASTIAN MUDERS

ONE OF THE most widespread criticisms against the employment of human dignity in bioethical debates is its supposed meaninglessness. This charge is understandable insofar as the concept of human dignity, taken in isolation, is hardly suitable to do any work in applied ethics. Instead, like other basic concepts in normative ethics (e.g., justice or virtue), the notion of human dignity first needs to be elaborated with the help of further notions before it can be brought to bear on specific cases.

Two of the most prominent attempts to undertake such an elaboration within the debate on assisted dying consist in interpreting dignity either in terms of autonomy or in terms of the value of human life. Interestingly, these conceptions are usually presented as competing; that is, either one spells out human dignity in terms of autonomy, or one explicates it in terms of the value of human life.

As an alternative, I offer what might be called a "combined approach," seeking to explicate dignity in terms of specific interpretations of both autonomy and life's value in a way that gives a *unique normative role* to both, and I argue that both are *compatible with each other*. This will help explain our complex attitudes toward various cases of assisted dying.

This chapter is structured as follows. In the first section, I explain my motivation for linking two important arguments in the debate on assisted death, the argument from autonomy and the argument from the value of life, to human dignity. Next, I provide two conceptions of dignity that can be used to enhance these arguments by being linked to specific interpretations of human beings' capacity for practical rationality. In a third step, I show how these dignity conceptions can be viewed in many cases as being compatible with one another. Finally, I apply these insights to cases of assisted death, arguing that both "dignity-enhanced" arguments can be recognized as valid without either having priority with respect to the other. Still, each one might be employed for turning the tide in favor of or against assisted death.

Two Arguments

Margaret Battin helpfully distinguishes five arguments in the debate on assisted death.[1] The argument from autonomy and the argument from mercy are used in favor of assisted death, whereas the argument from the integrity of the physician's profession, the slippery slope argument, and the argument from the special value of life are employed against it.

In what follows, I concentrate on the two arguments that are most frequently linked to human dignity—the argument from autonomy and the argument from the special value of life. Notably, both arguments do not merely question the moral legitimacy of *assisting* persons who seek their death but also question the act of willingly killing oneself, with or without assistance, *itself*. In contrast, the arguments from the integrity of the physician's profession and the argument from mercy primarily address the reasons that assisting persons have to help others kill themselves.

Furthermore, in contrast to the slippery slope argument, the arguments from autonomy and from the special value of life can be interpreted as principle-based: They are usually formulated by referring to general, situation-independent norms of conduct, the prohibition not to kill innocent human beings, and the norm to respect persons' autonomous choices. This does not preclude that they may have some exceptions, pointing to cases in which they are either overruled by competing principles or even "silenced" as moral considerations. Nevertheless, both formulate rules that share a wide scope of application: In general, innocent human life is to be protected, and in general, we ought to respect the decisions made by others.

In cases of assisted dying, both rules are often applicable. Consider the following two examples. In a first case, a teenager jumps to his death from a bridge after his favorite TV soap opera was canceled.[2] In a second case

---

[1] See Margaret Pabst Battin, "The Irony of Supporting Physician-Assisted Suicide: A Personal Account," *Medical Health Care and Philosophy* 13, no. 4 (2010): 403–411, 404.

[2] See Margaret Pabst Battin, *The Least Worth Death* (New York: Oxford University Press, 1994), 267. The case took place in Minnesota on August 23, 1979, when fifteen-year-old Eddie Seidel Jr. jumped from St. Paul's High Bridge after the cancelation of the TV series *Battlestar Galactica*.

reported by Ronald Dworkin, a seventy-six-year-old widow never left an intensive care unit after her open-heart operation, endured crisis after crisis and insisted to be resuscitated should she suffer respiratory arrest on her ventilator [3] Most people will judge the first case to be a meaningless tragedy that ought to be prevented because the aesthetical value of a soap opera cannot outweigh the value of the teenager's life. With respect to the second example, I take it that we are inclined to argue that what matters here are not considerations about the widow's own good or well-being but, rather, her autonomous wish to be resuscitated: If she had decided otherwise, not resuscitating her would have become equally mandatory for the hospital staff.

What makes the teenager's life, understood as part of his well-being, the decisive factor in the first case, regardless of whether he formed his decision to die autonomously or not? Why is this not so in the second case, in which the widow's autonomous decision is decisive? I suggest that human dignity might provide us with additional resources to provide an answer to these questions. Given that the idea of dignity is tightly linked to a value of persons, and given that persons are of central significance in modern ethics, linking autonomy or the value of human life to human dignity might provide additional reasons why we ought to respect them in ways that forbid or allow killing oneself. I unfold this connection in the following two sections, first for the argument from autonomy and then for the argument from the value of life.

Human Dignity and Autonomy

If one seeks to ground the normative force of the principle of autonomy in human dignity, a natural suggestion how to connect both is to examine conceptions of human dignity that are Kantian in spirit. Stephen Darwall has put forward an influential suggestion in his article "The Value of Autonomy and Autonomy of the Will" and other texts. His leading aim is to give substance to the idea that persons, by a sheer act of willing, can provide reasons for themselves and others: " 'Because I want it' can sometimes give one a reason for acting that is additional to the reasons for which one wants or wills."[4]

[3] See Ronald Dworkin, *Life's Dominion: An Argument about Abortion, Euthanasia, and Individual Freedom* (New York: Knopf, 1993), 186.
[4] Stephen Darwall, "Because I Want It," *Social Philosophy and Policy* 18, no. 2 (2001): 129–153, 130.

"Reasons for which one wants or wills" can be understood in terms of what Darwall calls the "Moorean picture." Following this picture, which Darwall traces back to Moorean (meta)ethics, what we ought to do is promote valuable states of affairs, possible world states whose value exists independently of our wants and gives everyone reasons to act in accordance with them. Here, our practical reason works much like its theoretical counterpart in allowing us to achieve an adequate representation of the normative world, which in turn allows us to see what we ought to do.

Darwall finds this picture too one-sided, as it overlooks a kind of "freedom that is distinctive of practical reason." For within the realm of theoretical reason, it is "not being logically open to reject the bearing of objective probability and truth on what to believe."[5] However, the same is not true for its practical counterpart: Here, an additional source of reasons can be found in a "capacity persons have to impose demands that are rooted in the authority of free and rational wills as such and thus in no value outside the will."[6]

One argument Darwall offers for the existence of this source of reasons is a modified version of Moore's famous open-question argument. With this argument, Moore wanted to show that for every suggestion for analyzing the concept of good with reference to non-normative properties, it is always possible to question whether something that possesses these non-normative properties is indeed good. Darwall makes a similar move with respect to Moore's claim that we can analyze what we ought to do in terms of what would be good to do. If we focus merely on reasons given by the objects of our desires, it quickly turns out that

> we can step back from any perspective given us even by our most critically informed desires and sensibly ask whether what we have reason to do is just to promote valuable states (as they will seem from our desires' perspective).[7]

Darwall presents the following example that suggests that the answer to this question is negative. A young woman is visiting her parents. They serve her broccoli, despite their knowledge of the daughter's aversion

---

[5] Stephen Darwall, "Moore, Normativity, and Intrinsic Value," *Ethics* 113, no. 3 (2003): 468–489, 471.

[6] Stephen Darwall, "The Value of Autonomy and Autonomy of the Will," *Ethics* 116, no. 2 (2006): 263–284, 264.

[7] Darwall, "Moore, Normativity, and Intrinsic Value," 485.

against this kind of food. Darwall invites us to imagine how the parents "urge her over her protests to 'eat her broccoli'" because they believe that this would best promote her welfare, and he asks what makes their action wrong. He maintains that their behavior's "objectionable character" is not best described as

> misdirected care or even negligently misdirected care. It is, rather, primarily a failure of respect, a failure to recognize the authority that persons have to demand, within certain limits, that they be allowed to make their own choices for themselves.[8]

This authority, Darwall believes, lies at the heart of the conception of the dignity of persons as Kantians conceive it. Dignity thus understood signifies a certain authority to make claims that deserve our normative attention independently of any supporting value-related considerations. Darwall calls this authority "autonomy as a claim or demand." This authority in turn is grounded in the nature of persons as free and rational beings, which possess a capacity Darwall calls "autonomy of the will."[9]

Without having the space to discuss Darwall's complex position in detail, the connection between his Kantian conception of dignity and the argument from autonomy should be clear enough: Under this interpretation, the argument from autonomy, which states that we should respect the autonomous decisions of others, refers to the specific kind of autonomy—autonomy as a claim or demand—Darwall has in mind. Choices that make use of this autonomy rooted in the nature of free beings can create an obligation for other people not to interfere with them even in light of conflicting considerations regarding the person's welfare.

Because the life of a person is relevant for her welfare—be it merely constitutive for other aspects of her welfare or be it a stand-alone element in it—one can see how this version of the argument from autonomy might be used to overcome conflicting considerations brought into play by the argument from the value of life. Before replacing the broccoli example with a case more suitable for the present discussion of suicide, however, let me first explore a different conception of human dignity that is often used to support the argument from the value of life.

---

[8] Darwall, "The Value of Autonomy," 268.
[9] Darwall, "The Value of Autonomy," 264.

Human Dignity and Life's Value

Like Darwall's Kantian conception of dignity, a competing conception linkable to the argument from the special value of life starts with the identification of certain capacities present in the bearers of human dignity. In addition, these capacities show a striking similarity to the ones mentioned by Darwall, if only in name. Whereas Darwall speaks of the capacity of free will that stems from the nature of persons as "free and rational beings," Patrick Lee and Robert George, two proponents of new natural law theory who are among the most prominent defenders of the (special) value of life, similarly refer to "natural capacities for conceptual thought, deliberation, and free choice" as the features that are responsible for the "personal dignity" possessed by all members of the human species.[10]

However, closer inspection reveals important differences in the understanding of these capacities. The capacity for conceptual thought allows human beings to "reflect back upon themselves and their place in reality; that is, they can attain an objective view, and they can attempt to be objective in their assessments and choices."[11] This description suggests a power of practical reason that is roughly analogous to theoretical reason in the way depicted by Darwall.

This impression is fostered when we turn our attention to the capacity for free choice. Following the new natural lawyers (NLL), a free choice is rational only when it is directed toward an alternative that presents itself as desirable or valuable in some form or another, *and* as long as no other considerations are recognizably better. By far not all choices qualify for this. Lee and George cite an example of house hunting and imagine two properties that are almost identical in their demanded features, save for one, which can only be found in the first residence: "In that situation, the second house cannot be chosen, since it has no distinctive attractiveness."[12]

Thus, in contrast to Darwall, rational free choice remains bound to the value of the objects of our choices. The capacities of conceptual thought and free choice, taken together under the heading of rationality, mark the decisive normative difference between human beings and other creatures, granting them their special status called "dignity." Because these

---

[10] Patrick Lee and Robert P. George, "The Nature and Basis of Human Dignity," *Ratio Juris* 21, no. 2 (2008): 173–193.

[11] Patrick Lee and Robert P. George, *Body–Self Dualism in Contemporary Ethics and Politics* (New York: Cambridge University Press, 2007), 56.

[12] Lee and George, *Body–Self Dualism*, 56. See also John Finnis, John Boyle, and Germain Grisez, *Nuclear Deterrence, Morality, and Realism* (Oxford: Clarendon, 1987), 258–259.

capacities are taken to be deeply rooted in human nature, a first interpretation of the argument from the special value of life suggests itself: If "human life" is read as "human existence," the principle underlying this argument commands us to treat human beings with special care in contrast to other entities.

Although I think that this interpretation is correct, it does not yet tell us what renders assisted death morally problematic. Because the capacities for conceptual thought and free choice not only dignify our existence in the first place but also allow us to recognize our special worth by having them, treating ourselves appropriately involves the proper exercise of these capacities; that is, we should freely direct our choices in ways that track the assessments given by our capacity for understanding of what is valuable—for us and others.

This reasoning allows the NLL to supplement the first interpretation with a second one. Here, "human life" is understood not as tantamount to the whole human person but, rather, as an important aspect of what is valuable for her. How can life be considered as valuable for human beings? Three options are available. First, human life might be of *overwhelming importance* for human beings, meaning that an action in which life is sacrificed for another part of someone's well-being can never be justified. This particularly strong interpretation has counterintuitive results: Some aspects of my well-being (e.g., unbearable pain) or of the well-being of others (e.g., the lives of my children) appear to justify the sacrifice of my life.

A second alternative regards life as *one final good among others*—one good among others that can be sought for its own sake—that can rationally be put into jeopardy only under two conditions: First, the life-threatening action must be directed toward another final good incomparable with the good of life, so that it cannot be judged *worse* than the life that would be sacrificed. Second, the realization of this second good must be pursued in a way that does not show any *disrespect* toward the value of life or any other final good damaged or lost in this enterprise. One shows disrespect toward a final good when one treats it as not valuable at all or less valuable than it really is. This interpretation is favored by the NLL, and they employ it to justify their prohibition of assisted dying.[13]

---

[13] For an interpretation of life's value along these lines and a rejection of the alternative to regard life as an absolute good, see John Keown, "Restoring the Sanctity of Life and Replacing the Caricature: A Reply to David Price," *Legal Studies* 26, no. 1 (2006): 109–119. NLL and other defenders of natural law ethics often use "basic," "intrinsic," or "fundamental" good, whereas

A third alternative (compatible with the second one) regards life as *constitutively valuable* by being a necessary ingredient in the goods that are of final value. Examples for such goods are the experience of joyfulness, the active engagement in valuable personal relationships, or, more generally, the appreciation of things that a person recognizes as objects of worthwhile activities. Again, to willfully ignore these available goods by killing oneself is rational only when doing so is the only possibility to realize another final good not worse than these, in a way that does not treat them as not valuable at all or as less valuable than they really are. This alternative alone will regard many cases of assisted dying as permissible (i.e., when none of the goods constituted by being alive are available anymore), so again the NLL usually focus on the second option.

The first interpretation and one or more versions of the second interpretation, taken together, generate the following reading for a dignity-enhanced argument from the special value of life: Assisted death is wrong when it involves an action that disrespects life as an important good of a bearer of human dignity, which in turn results in the death of the dignity bearer and subsequently in the blameworthy loss of her personal dignity, a value grounded in her rational capacities.

Two Kinds of Human Dignity or One?

Following this outline, it might be tempting to conclude that there are two distinct, even mutually excluding conceptions of the capacities termed "(practical) rationality" that are responsible for human dignity. Hence, the conceptions of human dignity that flow from this, and the norms that are justified by appealing to it, are also distinct. In what follows, I argue that this impression is false. Instead, we should regard both capacities as responsible for a single normative phenomenon called "dignity" that can give non-contradictory normative guidance for specific cases of assisted dying.

Let us begin with the claim that both ways of giving an account of our capacity of practical rationality are compatible with each other. Starting with Darwall's picture, he notably does not deny that at least *some* practical reasons are *not* given by the will of other agents but, rather, grounded in the features of non-personal entities. Moreover, he is cautious not to

---

I say "final" good; see Timothy D. J. Chappell, *Understanding Human Goods: A Theory of Ethics* (Edinburgh, UK: Edinburgh University Press, 1998), chap. 2.1–2.2.

claim that his account of human dignity is exhaustive: He only writes that his depiction of dignity as an authority that human beings possess as free and rational beings captures a "central component of our dignity" that is "part of the dignity of persons."[14]

Indeed, it seems plausible that an authority of the kind Darwall has in mind will hardly provide its bearer with normative directions all on its own. When giving his example of a sergeant who orders his platoon to fall in, Darwall highlights that for the sergeant's men, the command given has normative force whether nor not they believe that this order is supported by independent reasons.[15]

For the sergeant herself, however, this alone will not do. From her own perspective, she has the authority to set out a specific range of commands to those under her control; but this authority merely *permits* her to issue commands; it does not specify whether and when she should give them, nor what exact content they have. Thus, before she makes use of this right, she needs to look for further reasons she has to issue specific orders. Some of these might consist in other orders she received from her superior authority, but others might be good-based reasons. If she completely stops to take these further reasons into account and begins to issue commands at whim, her subordinates might legitimately begin to question her authority.

These reflections do no show that each exercise of the authority we possess as persons depends on preceding reasons of the Moorean sort. Still, they do indicate that there is nothing weird with the general idea that a legitimate use of one's authority might be subject to a requirement to take into account the good-based reasons one has for doing things. The assumption of such a requirement will presumably be more plausible if we conceive of an agent's autonomous wishes as "judgment-sensitive attitudes," as Scanlon calls them.[16] Also, the more there is at stake when making use of this authority—for the agent or others—the more the introduction of such a requirement seems to be justified. I return to this later.

For the moment, let us concentrate on a natural worry that will arise when we begin to regard the consideration of good-based reasons as a rational requirement for the rational exercise of personal authority. Given this requirement, there seems to be little or no room for the freedom to

---

[14] Stephen Darwall, "Respect and the Second-Person Standpoint," *Proceedings and Addresses of the American Philosophical Association* 78, no. 2 (2004): 43–59, 44; Darwall, "The Value of Autonomy," 268.

[15] See Stephen Darwall, *The Second-Person Standpoint* (Cambridge, Mass.: Harvard University Press, 2006), 12–13.

[16] Thomas M. Scanlon, *What We Owe to Each Other* (Cambridge, Mass.: Belknap, 1998), 20–21.

choose, which was part of the motivation that led Darwall to introduce reasons based on authority: It was precisely this lack of freedom that prompts his version of the open-question argument against the exclusivity of Moorean-style reasons in practical deliberation.

To respond to this concern, I suggest that not only should defenders of authority-based reasons allow good-based reasons as further elements within their deliberative framework; proponents of good-based reasons should also conversely grant authority-based reasons a role within their pluralistic framework of what is good for human beings.

Let us return to Darwall's broccoli example. The parents' behavior obviously suffers from their misjudgment about the influence of broccoli on their daughter's health. But imagine they were correct. How could a good-based theory of reasons of the kind defended by natural law theorists mark the parents' behavior as paternalistic in the pejorative sense, no matter how healthy we conceive the broccoli to be? The usual move for NLL here is to identify a further good incomparable with the former—the good of integrity, or even autonomy[17]—and then to claim that the daughter's wish not to be spoon-fed by her parents can be interpreted not as denying the status of healthiness as a good but, rather, that in the situation at hand, securing this other good is of more importance to her.[18] Given that the good of autonomy is indeed as final as the good of (one's) health, and given the incomparability of both goods, the NLL might argue that contrary to the parents' assumptions, it is false that improving their daughter's health is *a better thing to do* than allowing her to make her own decisions.

But let us suppose again that the parents agree with this. They might admit that the superiority of their own value considerations is only justified from the perspective of their own preferences. Still, they add, even from their daughter's normative point of view, promoting healthiness is at least *not objectively worse* than allowing the daughter to realize (an instance of) the good she prefers.[19] So why should the adult daughter's preferences count for more than their own?

---

[17] See Philip E. Devine, *Natural Law Ethics* (Westport, Conn.: Greenwood Press, 2000), 71, 73–74; Alfons Gómez-Lobo, *Morality and the Human Goods: An Introduction to Natural Law Ethics* (Washington, D.C.: Georgetown University Press, 2002), 23–24.

[18] The possibility to let subjective preferences decide in these situations is described in John Finnis, *Natural Law and Natural Rights*, 2nd ed. (Oxford: Oxford University Press, 2011), 93.

[19] For the possibility to make an "at least not worse than" claim between incomparable goods, see Mark C. Murphy, *Natural Law and Practical Rationality* (New York: Cambridge University Press, 2001), 205–206.

Because all value-based considerations have been exhausted, it seems natural to look somewhere else for a further source of reasons that would explain our judgment against the parents' behavior. Following Darwall,[20] it might be helpful to note a normative shift in the parents' relationship to their daughter as a little child and as an adult. When she was young, their care was legitimately oriented toward her welfare. As parents, they now still care much about their daughter's well-being, but in contrast to her being a child, they now have to give her preferences in her own matters additional weight against their own wishes, thereby honoring the rationality and freedom she has developed to decide for herself. This, of course, is a person-bound authority of the kind Darwall has in mind: No matter how much weight the parents give their own preferences regarding what is objectively good for their daughter, these concerns are (in this case) silenced as reasons by the daughter's authority of her own preferences regarding what is actually also objectively good for her.

Thus, although not all instances of practical deliberation call for our capacity to exercise a kind of freedom that gives our wants a decisive normative weight, many will. Conversely, although not all instances of practical deliberation make it necessary that the options among which one freely chooses are themselves oriented toward the good, many will. So, in contexts in which our capacity to orient ourselves toward what is good and our capacity to choose freely both come into play, respecting the dignity they give its bearer will translate into respecting the ways in which the bearer uses both.

Human Dignity and Assisted Death

The question I pursue now is whether and how both capacities are relevant in the case of suicide. This in turn will allow us to give a first assessment of the legitimacy and limits of the arguments from autonomy and from the value of life in cases of assisted death.

Let us start with the deliberation of someone considering suicide. I previously stated that apart from the question of whether the fact that I simply want to do something *always* has some normative weight on its own, we must ask whether this weight is sufficient to counter good-based reasons even in cases in which much is at stake for the agent (or others). Consider my (autonomous) wish for an ice cream when I am

---

[20] See Darwall, "The Value of Autonomy," 267.

walking through a park. It is plausible to assume that under standard conditions, I do not first have to examine whether my wish is adequately supported by good-based reasons; I might take my wish for an ice cream as already authoritative for me to buy one (and for others not to interfere with my plan). Contrast this with my wish to die. Given the difficult-to-overestimate influence my death has on my overall well-being, if any case is suited to endorse a requirement to take into account the good-based reasons I have to kill myself, then this one is. To follow a mere wish to bring about my death without considering whether I have reasons to do so seems like irrational behavior of a kind that is difficult to exceed in irrationality.

It might seem that a stand-alone wish to die, if it is truly *mine*, not only has normative weight but also can be decisive in determining what my current well-being consists in. So far, I have assumed that autonomous wishes may or may not stand opposed to good-based reasons as depicted by the Moorean picture. But it might be argued that what is good for me and the reasons I get from these facts are determined, at least to a large extent, from what I autonomously prefer.[21] On one influential account developed by Wayne Sumner, the contents of a person's well-being can be equated with her authentic endorsement of them, which includes their experiencing them as satisfying or fulfilling.[22] Their endorsement in turn is authentic when based on preferences that are well-informed and autonomous,

---

[21] This way of introducing the argument assumes a specific answer to the question how an autonomous desire and a free will are ontologically related to each other. We might assume that an autonomous desire is constituted by a metaphysically free will of mine—that is, a desire that has my own non-determined will as its causal starting point. Natural Law defenders usually have this conception in mind when speaking about free will (Joseph M. Boyle, Germain Grisez, and Olaf Tollefsen, *Free Choice: A Self-Referential Argument* (Notre Dame, Ind.: University of Notre Dame Press, 1976)). Alternatively, one might believe that a free will is constituted by an autonomous desire, where the latter has to fulfill a set of criteria that do not presuppose the existence of a metaphysically free will. A third possibility would be to keep the concept of a free will and the concept of an autonomous desire entirely separate: Following this alternative, it would make sense to say that the reasons I get from a (metaphysically) free will are one thing, whereas the reasons delivered by the fact that my desires fulfill certain criteria and thus count as autonomous are quite another. In the following discussion of the argument, I assume that either the second alternative is true or that the third option is correct in a way that only these (metaphysically) free choices provide the agents and others with reasons that are based on autonomous desires.

[22] See W. L. Sumner, *Welfare, Happiness, and Ethics* (Oxford: Clarendon, 1996), 139, 171–172. I here take Sumner's theory as my example because it combines many of the advantages of the two leading subjectivist theories of well-being: hedonism and the desire-fulfillment theory. Still, the distinction between autonomous and non-autonomous desires is a standard move within preference-based welfare theories; see Chris Heathwood, "Desire-Fulfillment Theory," in *The Routledge Handbook of Philosophy of Well-Being*, ed. Guy Fletcher (London: Routledge, 2016): 135–147, 142–143.

where the former is itself analyzed as a function of what the person auton-omously would want to know.[23]

The criteria Sumner employs to qualify wants as autonomous are them-selves not dependent on the good-based reasons an agent has. He suggests a mixture of "coherentist" (where what matters are the logical relations between different sorts of preferences) and "responsiveness-to-reasoning" criteria (where what matters is the agent's formal capacity to evaluate her preferences).[24] This way of empowering autonomy regarding the range of reasons it provides provokes a worry that mirrors the concern Darwall expresses when wondering about the possibility that all reasons are good-based: When deliberating about what we ought to do in light of our own good, are we really just trying to find out what we *really* (freely) want?

Battin's previously mentioned example of the teenager who jumped to his death after his favorite TV soap opera was canceled suggests a nega-tive answer. The particularities of this case naturally point to the victim's young age and that his irrational behavior might well be explained as a case of non-autonomous decision-making. Although this might do justice to the case at hand, one wonders whether our judgment regarding the rea-sonableness of the teenager's action should change if we presume that he was deciding autonomously according to the standards a preference-based theory of well-being is able to offer. I believe our judgment should remain the same, for the *explanandum* remains unchanged: Sacrificing one's life in the face of the (henceforth absent) aesthetical value of a soap opera is simply an unreasonable thing to do.

Switching back to the deliberation of the person seeking suicide, I con-clude that the mere fact that her wish is autonomous cannot provide her with sufficient reasons that, from the perspective of her well-being, she ought to follow. Whatever the exact normative weight this fact bears on her decision, there are other considerations to which she should pay atten-tion, namely the good-based reasons that speak in favor or against her wish. However, if she does pay attention to them[25] but still autonomously

---

[23] See Sumner, *Welfare*, 160.

[24] See Sumner, *Welfare*, 167–171. I take the labels and the characterization for these accounts from Sarah Buss, "Personal Autonomy," *The Stanford Encyclopedia of Philosophy (Winter 2016 Edition)* (2016), https://plato.stanford.edu/archives/win2016/entries/personal-autonomy, accessed January 7, 2017. "Formal capacity" here refers to measures for securing autonomous deliberation that do not include the content of preference-independent reasons an agent has.

[25] In my understanding, "paying attention to the reasons" minimally requires me to recognize and accept the normative implications that the relevant good-related considerations have for my decision. That even recognizing *all* such implications is compatible with the exercise of my authority as a free and rational being was one upshot of the previous section. Given the relevance of good-based reasons for my well-being for which I have just argued, it could be tempting to

decides against them, we should still say that her choice has *some* dignity and deserves *some* respect[26]: This is the lesson to be drawn from Darwall's suggestions. It just seems that at least in matters of life and death, this respect does not extend to the overall assessment of what the suicidal person ought to do.

Or does it? Changing the perspective from a suicidal person's own deliberative standpoint to the practical standpoint of others, this may be doubted. Granted, a person's well-being, if authoritative for anyone, is providing *her* with reasons of what she ought to do. Still, one can legitimately question whether it gives *others* permission to urge her to bring it about.[27] On the other hand, a person's autonomous wish does give others reasons to respect it, as Darwall's broccoli case has made clear.

Imagine now, however, that, in a variation of this case, when the daughter is visiting her parents, they somehow come to know that she has suicidal intentions. Furthermore, suppose that the daughter's reasons are similar to those of the teenager discussed previously. It is difficult to believe that the parents would be engaged in wrongful paternalism if they urge her to give up her plans. Given their emotional ties with her, we plausibly expect that they care *about what happens to her* because they care *for her:* Due to their love for her, they see her as a person worthy of their consideration.

This reasoning points to a normative bridge between the reasons a person has to care for her well-being and the reasons anyone may have for doing so—a bridge that is assumed within both conceptions of dignity under consideration. Darwall presents a particularly strong interpretation of this bridge, for he identifies "what it is for something to be good for someone" with "what it is for something that one should desire it for someone *for her sake*, that is, insofar as one cares for her."[28] Care in turn is characterized as a kind of response by the caring person that is directed toward the person as someone who the caring person experiences as valuable in

---

question the autonomy of persons who miss important good-related considerations relevant for their decision, for they do *not* seem to be "well-informed" in one sense. This, however, just highlights the fact that to prevent the collapse of responsiveness-to-reasoning accounts into responsiveness-to-reason theories, their notion of autonomy has to allow for this kind of shortcoming.

[26] I take the expression "some dignity" from Nussbaum's remark that human beings are "creatures of whom it is true that the fact that they reach out for something has itself some importance, some dignity" (Martha Craven Nussbaum, *Women and Human Development: The Capabilities Approach* (New York: Cambridge University Press, 2001), 146).

[27] See Guy Fletcher, "A Fresh Start for the Objective-List Theory of Well-Being," *Utilitas* 25, no. 2 (2013): 206–220, 210.

[28] Stephen Darwall, *Welfare and Rational Care* (Princeton, N.J.: Princeton University Press, 2002), 8–9. Darwall attributes similar ideas to Elizabeth Anderson and David Velleman. See note 35.

an agent-neutral sense.[29] In other words, it is *the cared person's value as experienced* that leads the caring person to have the desire for the cared person being in certain states, and these states are constitutive for the cared person's well-being.[30]

Similarly, natural law theorists often seek to identify what is beneficial for persons—a content they usually explicate in perfectionist terms—as "intrinsic" to them, by being related to the agent-neutral value they have as persons. On that view, harming a person's well-being is harming the person, whereas promoting it is promoting the person by making her being more fulfilling.[31] Thus, in these theories, as in Darwall's, "the locus of value is the persons themselves."[32] As elaborated in the penultimate section, this value is called "dignity" by the NLL, and it is grounded in rational capacities that make human beings persons.

Darwall does not call this value "dignity."[33] He speaks about a person's "worth" as the evaluative endpoint for reasons of care, thus establishing "caring" as a distinct way of valuing someone for her own sake *besides* "respect." This is partly because he reserves the notion of dignity for a different kind of normative phenomenon explored in the second section: the authority persons possess to create reasons for themselves and others, whose resulting claims demand our respect. Another reason stems from his belief that although "respect for one's dignity is something anyone can demand, . . . this is not so with sympathetic concern . . . for one's welfare."[34] I return to this issue later. Let me first note that classificatory considerations and dangers of confusion aside, there seems to me apt reason to call a conception of the person's "worth" that brings its contents into close relationship with the intrinsic value of a person her "dignity." David Velleman has embarked on this path by suggesting that the value of a person that is not a value *for* him, but *in* him, is what the dignity of a person consists in.[35]

---

[29] See Darwall, *Welfare*, 71.

[30] Moreover, once someone has recognized a person's value, it works as a normative reason for her to care for the person even when she does not experience it anymore. See Darwall, *Welfare*, 72.

[31] See Murphy, *Natural Law*, 187–190, with further references. I think it is no coincidence that Darwall's own view regarding the contents of a human being's welfare can also be characterized as a kind of perfectionism.

[32] Lee and George, "The Nature and Basis of Human Dignity," 181.

[33] But see Darwall, *Welfare*, 78.

[34] Darwall, *The Second Person Standpoint*, 128.

[35] See David Velleman, "A Right of Self-Termination?", *Ethics* 109, no. 3 (1999): 606–628, 611, 613. As Velleman notes, he is equating "the value that we appreciate in caring about a person with the value that we appreciate, somewhat differently, in respecting that person in the Kantian sense." Darwall would deny this equation, whereas I suggest to extent it to *both* senses of dignity as an

Regardless of how plausible the *general* connection between the intrinsic value a person has due to her rational nature and her well-being might be, at least one aspect of the latter seems highly relevant for the former: her life. Given that a person's existence presupposes her biological existence, her death will often be something we have reason to avoid for the person's sake. Furthermore, if there is an aspect of care that, *pace* Darwall, anyone can reasonably demand from us, then it is our care in relation to actions that have a direct influence on someone's death.

The caring concern of the daughter's parents will lead to their justified resistance to accept her wish to die caused by her disappointment at the cancelation of a soap opera. I believe, moreover, that we do not have to have a special relationship with someone in order to be under the obligation to be wary when an omission or action of ours can foreseeably help to bring about someone's death. After all, even acts of ours that greatly influence the well-being of creatures with a non-personal nature to a lesser degree stand under such an obligation: If I can easily prevent the torture of a cat, I surely have very good reasons to do so.

Cats are not human beings, and human beings (at least most of them) are persons—that is, free and rational beings. Although their ability for free choice and the authority this gives them for creating reasons that guide their own as well others' behavior does make a difference in how they should be treated even for the sake of their well-being, it does not follow, I have argued, that these reasons always outweigh the reasons we have to care about their well-being. Indeed, they will often not outweigh them in matters of life and death, such as when someone is seeking suicide. Because facts about a person's well-being are not reducible to what she autonomously and freely wants, what a person really wishes for herself and what is good for her can diverge (although they do not have to).

Indeed, the fact that the two may not diverge allows for an important qualification regarding what one should want for her *for her own sake*. If we accept the NNL claim that a person may have to choose between incomparable goods when acting on behalf of her own welfare, it might be that even the most reasonable and faultless reflection of what is good for someone can lead to different conclusions if drawn by different persons (or the same person at different times). This explains why, in Dworkin's example of the widow who insisted on being resuscitated, the old woman might rightfully value her life even in her miserable condition but could

---

authority and as a value. Notably, Velleman also presents his argument in the context of the debate on physician-assisted suicide.

equally well have chosen to spare herself further suffering and not to be resuscitated as she finally suffered respiratory arrest on her ventilator. Given that her autonomous wish has normative weight on its own, an equally well-founded conclusion her relatives might have arrived at—that not resuscitating her will leave her no worse off than doing so—cannot outweigh the widow's own reasoning.

Moreover, depending on how much weight we give a person's autonomous preferences, even if a terminally ill person freely opts for an alternative that is worse with respect to her well-being than another one also available to her, this can give decisive reason for others to respect her wishes. Imagine that a heavily suffering person faces the choice between terminal sedation and euthanasia. The latter would suffice to prevent her from further suffering, and we might think that, even in this state, her life has special value, being still "human through and through."[36] Although choosing euthanasia thus makes this patient objectively worse off, one might argue that the remaining value of her life as such—putting aside the constitutive value it has for many other things the patient will not be able to realize when being terminally sedated—is not important enough to outweigh the reason to respect her autonomous choice for assisted dying.

Conclusion

In this chapter, I have suggested that two conceptions of dignity that are often treated as competing can be interpreted as being compatible with each other: first, dignity as an authority persons possess as free and rational beings, an authority that allows them to create reasons for themselves and others; and second, dignity as an intrinsic value free and rational beings possess as subjects that can be guided by what is objectively good—for themselves or others.

These conceptions can be employed in the arguments from autonomy and from the value of life, which both play an important role in the debate on assisted death. Thus employed, the argument from autonomy states that we ought to respect a person's dignity by giving due weight to her authority

---

[36] John Finnis, "A Philosophical Case against Euthanasia," in *Euthanasia Examined*, ed. John Keown (Cambridge: Cambridge University Press, 1995), 23–35, 30–31. That a human life "is not partly carrot-life and partly cat-life" to which former state it is reducible when being terminally sedated (or in a persistent vegetative state) strikes me as correct: Even then (and also after their death), we still must treat human beings in these conditions appropriately and differently from how we treat carrots—for example, by not humiliating them and not abusing them.

to decide for herself in matters of life and death, albeit this authority does not outweigh all considerations that speak in favor or against her wish to die. Within the range of a person's own authority, one must respect her decision with regard to her own acts, even when, due to reasons of care, we have good reason to want her to choose differently. On the other hand, the dignity-enhanced argument from the value of life demands from us that we act in accordance with the intrinsic worth we have as creatures who can be guided by what is desirable independently from our preferences. To respect this capacity means to give good-based reasons the appropriate normative weight and not to give our own wants undue normative weight.

I have left open the question what exact normative weight our free decision possesses relative to the demands of competing good-based reasons. Still, I have claimed that in matters of life and death, one cannot do *without* the latter kind of considerations. Also, I have given no specific answer regarding the question which kind of value we should ascribe to human life—absolute value, final value, or constitutive value. Although I admit that this would be necessary for a complete philosophical case for or against assisted dying, it will not touch directly on the conception of human dignity defended here; if part of our dignity consists in our capacity to follow what we recognize as good for us (and others), what is good for us (and others) must be clarified by a convincing theory of well-being. Still, I have pointed out that our well-being cannot be adequately captured solely by what we autonomously want. Also, what makes our well-being normatively relevant for us and others is at least partly constituted by the intrinsic value we enjoy as beings endowed with certain capacities.[37]

---

[37] I am very grateful to Holger Baumann, Carina Fourie, Christoph Halbig, Philipp Schwind, and the participants of two research seminars at the Center for Ethics of the University of Zurich for helpful comments and feedback on previous versions of this chapter.

CHAPTER 9 | Dignity and Assisted Dying
What Kant Got Right (and Wrong)

MICHAEL CHOLBI

WERE IMMANUEL KANT able to eavesdrop on contemporary debates about the morality of assisted dying, he would likely be puzzled by how his moral philosophy is invoked. On the one hand, many advocates for a moral right to assisted dying hold that individuals are entitled to a "death with dignity." On this view, autonomous rational agents are sometimes morally entitled to end their lives when they judge that they are better off dying sooner rather than later. To bar physicians (or others) from providing assistance in dying would therefore be a wrongful infringement on an individual's autonomy and his or her right to pursue a dignified death. The 1997 "Philosophers' Brief" on behalf of the legal permissibility of assisted dying typifies this perspective:

> Each individual has a right to make the "most intimate and personal choices central to personal dignity and autonomy." That right encompasses the right to exercise some control over the time and manner of one's death. . . . A person's interest in following his own convictions at the end of life is so central a part of the more general right to make "intimate and personal choices" for himself that a failure to protect that particular interest would undermine the general right altogether.[1]

Kant would no doubt hear in such appeals echoes of his own characteristic moral doctrines—in particular, that because rational agents are to be

---

[1] Ronald Dworkin et al., "Assisted Suicide: The Philosophers' Brief," *New York Review of Books*, March 27, 1997. Available at http://www.nybooks.com/articles/archives/1997/mar/27/assisted-suicide-the-philosophers-brief.

respected as ends in themselves, we are obligated to defer to their choices regarding their own welfare.

On the other hand, an eavesdropping Kant[2] would almost certainly be shocked to see himself depicted as an ally of a moral right to end one's life with the assistance of others. For while Kant had little to say specifically about assistance in dying, he was emphatic in his denunciations of suicide. In his *Lectures on Ethics*, for example, Kant says that those who engage in suicide treat themselves as little better than animals and should be seen as "carrion" (LE 27:372) with no "inner worth" (LE 27:344). And although we ought to sympathize with those suffering from "grief, worry, and depression," suicide itself should inspire "revulsion" or "hate" (LE 27:372–375). As discussed later, Kant would be particularly puzzled by invocations of "dignity" as a moral basis for the right to end one's life. For in Kant's eyes, human dignity is precisely what morally rules out such a right. And presumably, if Kant believed that there is no general right to end one's life, he would also have believed that there is no right to others' assistance in doing so.

Our aim here is to sort out, historically and philosophically, what Kant's understanding of dignity implies about assisted dying. Unlike many commentators, I am fairly sympathetic to Kant's argument that suicide violates duties to oneself and specifically that the general right to make choices regarding our own welfare is coherent only if we also are subject to a duty to preserve the rational agency exercised in making such choices. Nevertheless, I contend that Kant's argument does not establish an obligation to forego suicide (and hence, an obligation on the part of others not to assist in suicide) in each and every case. Although Kant's ethics, and his notion of dignity in particular, cannot be deployed to defend a broad permission for suicide akin to that favored by the "death with dignity" movement, it also does not entail as restrictive a stance on morally permissible suicide, or on assisted dying, as Kant might have supposed.

To home in on this modified Kantian position, we first need an accurate grasp of Kant's notion of dignity. To that end, the first section situates

[2] References to Kant's works are as follows: Parenthetical references are to the *Lectures on Ethics* (LE), *Metaphysics of Morals* (G), and *Groundwork of the Metaphysics of Morals* (MM). Citations are to volume and page numbers in the Berlin Akademie Edition of Kant's works (1901–). Translations of LE are from Immanuel Kant, *Lectures on Ethics*, ed. J. B. Schneewind, trans. P. Heath (Cambridge: Cambridge University Press, 2001). Translations of G and MM are from Immanuel Kant, *Practical Philosophy*, ed. and trans. M. J. Gregor (Cambridge: Cambridge University Press, 1996).

Kant's notion in relation to other historically prominent notions of dignity. The next section outlines how Kant deploys his notion of dignity in his arguments for a fairly stringent duty of self-preservation and indicates how this duty entails the wrongfulness of assisted dying. Then, I defend Kant's understanding of dignity and how it generates a duty of self-preservation against contemporary Kantians who invoke dignity in defense of assisted dying. The following sections identify two kinds of "hopeless" situations that fall outside the scope of Kant's arguments for the moral impermissibility of suicide and assisted dying. I thus conclude that although Kant's arguments against a right to assisted dying are formidable and arguably rest on a more defensible conception of dignity than that used by putatively Kantian defenders of "death with dignity," the best version of Kant's position does not absolutely preclude assisted dying.

Dignity, Kantian and Otherwise

As Michael Rosen[3] has documented, dignity has had different meanings throughout its history. Let us therefore catalog various historically prominent understandings of dignity so as to pinpoint what distinguishes Kant's notion of dignity from rival understandings.

First, in some traditions, dignity is an attribute belonging only to certain noteworthy persons. The ancient Romans, for instance, associated *dignitas* with royalty or other high social rank. Those with dignity were thereby owed a measure of deference or esteem. The Romans would thus likely be taken aback by the notion of dignity articulated in the United Nations' *Universal Declaration of Human Rights*, wherein "all members of the human family" have "inherent dignity" or "worth."[4]

In contrast, on Kant's understanding of dignity, it is possessed by all practically rational agents. Individuals with what Kant calls "humanity" are able to choose both the ends they pursue and the means best suited to the realization of their ends. In so doing, according to Kant, practically rational agents exhibit the capacity to choose on the basis of rational principles or, in Kant's own vernacular, to give themselves a "law" for rational action. It is this capacity for rational lawgiving that grounds Kantian

---

[3] Michael Rosen, *Dignity: Its History and Meaning* (Cambridge, Mass.: Harvard University Press, 2012).

[4] United Nations, *Universal Declaration of Human Rights* (New York: United Nations, 1948), Preamble. Available at http://www.un.org/en/universal-declaration-human-rights, accessed November 14, 2016.

dignity.[5] Kant speaks of the "dignity of a rational being, who obeys no law other than that which he himself at the same time gives" (G 4:434) and of our capacity for "lawgiving itself" that "must for that very reason have a dignity" (G 4:436; see also G 4:439). For Kant, "autonomy," or our capacity to rationally choose—and act on the basis of—principles, is "the ground of the dignity of human nature and of every rational nature" (G 4:436). These rational capacities are not the province of the few, according to Kant. One need not be well born or a "dignitary" in order to have these elementary rational capacities of choice and action. Kantian dignity is thus effectively *universal*, the possession of all beings with practically rational capacities.

Second, some moral traditions follow Kant in holding that, for example, all human individuals have dignity, but they maintain that dignity itself is variegated so that not all such individuals have it in the same manner or to the same degree. Within Roman Catholic thinking, for example, all humans possess dignity, but the specific nature or magnitude of one's dignity depends on one's social role. Rosen summarizes the Roman Catholic stance as follows:

> All members of society have dignity, but their dignity consists in the role that is appropriate to their station within a hierarchical social order, one in which some are "nobler than others." Instead of sharing in equal dignity, the orders of society should differ in "dignity, rights, and power."[6]

On this conception of dignity, the dignity of priests differs from that of the laity, that of men differs from that of women, and so on. However, Kant's conception of dignity is *unified*. There is but one species of dignity, and all those with dignity possess it in the same manner and to the same degree. The dignity of a king neither exceeds nor is exceeded by the dignity of a pauper. Dignity is thus *equal* in its distribution.

Another distinguishing feature of Kant's conception of dignity is that it is *unmerited*. On some understandings of dignity, it is ascribed to those with a high level of moral character or wherewithal. Friedrich Schiller, for instance, thought of dignity as a "mastery of instinct by moral force." For

---

[5] Kant also associates dignity with morality or our capacity to be moral (G 4:425, G 4:435, G 4:440). However, these passages can plausibly be read as affirming the claim that dignity rests on our capacities for practical rationality. See Michael Cholbi, *Understanding Kant's Ethics* (Cambridge: Cambridge University Press, 2016), 111–112.

[6] Rosen, *Dignity: Its History and Meaning,* 49.

Schiller, the dignified person exerts a form of self-control over morally recalcitrant desires and thereby acts rightly.[7] Kant agrees with Schiller that a person deserves special moral credit when she resists desires that incline her to act immorally. Hence, our dignity is most plainly in view when we act morally. (G 4:435, MM 6:405) Nevertheless, he did not share with Schiller the belief that dignity is any type of moral accomplishment. For Kant, dignity is neither earned through morally praiseworthy action nor relinquished through morally blameworthy actions. Even the condemned murderer, Kant argues, retains dignity that precludes our justifiably torturing him, humiliating him, and so on (MM 6:333).

In a similar vein, some conceptions of dignity view it as a property of a person's bearing or demeanor. A person who exhibits steadfastness, independence, or tranquility, especially when confronting great adversity, is thereby dignified. This is one plausible way to gloss what advocates of assisted dying have in mind when they speak of a death "with dignity": a death in which a person is not racked with pain and able to keep his perceptual and cognitive faculties about him.[8] Kant would certainly agree that some behaviors we exhibit when under physical or mental strain are *contrary* to our dignity. He claims that "complaining and whining, even crying out in bodily pain, is unworthy" of beings with dignity (MM 6:436). But in such instances, it is the antecedent fact that we have dignity that makes it morally unseemly to behave in these ways. Again, we do not acquire dignity by behaving in dignified ways, nor do we lose it by behaving in undignified ways. Our dignity, Kant says, is not dependent on our actions or behavior and is in fact "*inalienable*" (MM 6:436).

These attributes of Kant's conception of dignity—that dignity is universal, unified, equal, and inalienable—go some way in vindicating Kant's claim to be the "father of the modern concept of human dignity."[9] For we see in Kant's conception of dignity a deeply egalitarian moral ethos at work. Dignity is a kind of high status, according to Kant, but one that elevates each and every human rational agent to that same high status. Kant would thus find the United Nations *Declaration*'s understanding of dignity—that because all "human beings are born free and equal in dignity"

---

[7] Friedrich Schiller, *On Grace and Dignity*, trans. G. Gregory (Washington, D.C.: Schiller Institute, [1793] 1992).

[8] Jyl Gentzler, "What Is a Death with Dignity?", *Journal of Medicine and Philosophy* 28 (2003): 461–462.

[9] Christopher McCrudden, "Human Dignity and Judicial Interpretation of Human Rights," *European Journal of International Law* 19 (2008): 655–724.

and "endowed with reason," they are thereby entitled to basic "rights and freedoms . . . without distinction of any kind"[10]—highly congenial.

Dignity, Price, and the Logic of Suicide

As noted previously, whereas many contemporary advocates of assisted dying understand dignity as licensing a right to choose one's own death, Kant clearly understood dignity as a source of duties to self—duties that prohibit the intentional taking of one's own life. The source of their dispute stems from the fact that, for Kant, dignity is not only a property that practically rational agents have. It is also a measure or kind of value, to be distinguished from *price*:

> Everything has either a *price* or a *dignity*. What has a price can be replaced by something as its *equivalent*; what on the other hand is raised above all price and therefore admits of no equivalent has dignity. . . . That which constitutes the condition under which alone something can be an end in itself has not merely a relative worth, that is, a price, but an inner worth, that is, *dignity*. (G 4:434–435)

Priceable goods, Kant claims, are fungible: It is both possible and morally permissible to exchange such goods for one another. We do so whenever we exchange material goods, sell our labor to one another, or conduct monetary transactions. Goods with a price are valuable either as means to the attainment of our chosen ends or because they are among our chosen ends. In contrast, that which has dignity, Kant claims, is an "end in itself" with "inner worth," not to be traded for priceable goods or for other goods with dignity. According to Kant, whatever has dignity has an "unconditional" and "incomparable" worth, a worth not commensurate with the "relative worth" of any priceable good (G 4:436). In conjunction with Kant's account of what has dignity (discussed previously), this taxonomy of value implies that rational agency is a distinctive good such that we are not morally entitled to attach a price to it or to trade it for what has price. Dignity is that through which rational agents are elevated "above all other beings in the world that are not human beings," beings that may permissibly be treated as "things." Rational agency must therefore be treated as an end in itself rather than merely as a means (MM 6:462). To sell a

---

[10] United Nations, *Universal Declaration of Human Rights*, articles 1 and 2.

human being into slavery, for example, is at odds with her dignity, for one is thereby limiting a person's liberty, and encumbering her rational agency, in exchange for money, a merely priceable good. Slave sales thus wrongfully treat an end in itself as a commodity to be used for furthering of others' goals or purposes.

But (Kant argues) self-killing is not fundamentally different from selling a person into slavery, inasmuch as when a person aims to end her life, she aims to destroy her own rational agency so as to further *her own* purposes. In so doing, a person wrongfully treats her rational agency as a means to her own happiness rather than (as the dignity of our rational agency demands) treating her rational agency as an end in itself: "A human being cannot be used merely as a means by any human being (either by others or *even by himself*) but must always be used at the same time as an end" (MM 6:462, emphasis added). Hence, to end one's life because doing so will, in one's own judgment, make for a better or happier life overall is to subordinate one's rational agency, which (again) has incomparably valuable dignity, to one's happiness, a "discretionary" good that merely has price. "Disposing of oneself as a mere means to some discretionary end is debasing" to our rational agency (MM 6:423) and contrary to our dignity. In effect then, Kant viewed suicide as practically contradictory—as an exercise of one's rational agency in which one destroys the very agency that grounds the value of one's choices in the first place (G 4:435). Suicide is thus at odds with "the first, though not the principal, duty of a human being to himself as an animal being"—the duty of self-preservation (MM 6:422).[11]

Before considering how Kant's anti-suicide argument denies a right to assisted dying, a few observations regarding the distinctive features of Kant's anti-suicide argument are in order.

First, note that Kant's opposition to suicide largely makes calculations of future happiness irrelevant to the moral justifiability of suicide. He is largely untroubled about whether an act of suicide is in fact prudent. Rather, his argument is meant to show that an individual's happiness simply cannot justify suicide:

Neither the greatest advantages, nor the highest degree of well-being, nor the most excruciating pains and even irremediable bodily sufferings can

---

[11] Here, I set aside the argument for a duty of self-preservation that Kant provides in the *Groundwork* (4:422), appealing to the alleged inability of a maxim permitting suicide from "self-love" to be consistently universalized. Few commentators find it compelling and many believe it lacks a proper basis in Kant's own ethical thinking. For further discussion, see Cholbi, *Understanding Kant's Ethics*, 184.

give a man the authority to take his own life, to escape from anguish and enter earlier upon a hoped-for higher happiness. (LE 27:628)

Second, Kant is also unconcerned with whether suicidal acts violate duties to others. Although his moral theory does not rule out that possibility (MM 6:423–424), Kant understands self-preservation as a duty we owe to ourselves. Thus, irrespective of whether a suicidal act wrongs others, it nevertheless violates a duty we owe ourselves as rational beings.

Finally, as the previous discussion of Kant's understanding of dignity underscores, the duty not to take one's own life is one that applies to us simply insofar as we are rational beings. Hence, all beings with dignity (i.e., all practically rational beings) have an obligation to forego suicide. Kant's duty does not make provisions for special pleading on behalf of the well born, those with particular social statuses, and so on.

One might assume that there is a direct logical path from Kant's moral opposition to suicide to a similar moral rejection of assisted dying. After all, if ending one's own life is wrong, and aiding another person in committing a moral wrong is itself wrong, then presumably Kant would hold that aiding another person in ending her life is wrong. There is, however, one complication here. The Kantian duty of self-preservation is classified as a duty of virtue rather than a duty of right (MM 6:329). A duty of right is one we can be compelled to fulfill via "external" compulsion or coercion. The duty not to steal, for example, is a duty individuals can be compelled to fulfill by threats of legal punishment. The duty of self-preservation, in contrast, is one we fulfill only when we not only keep ourselves alive but also do so because self-preservation is among the ends we endorse. But, Kant argues, although others can compel us to act in particular ways, they cannot compel us to act in those ways on the basis of particular ends or reasons. Our ends or reasons are wholly our own. The fulfillment of our duties to self is thus the result of "free self-constraint" (MM 6:382). Strictly speaking, then, the duty of self-preservation and, therefore, the duty not to take one's own life are not enforceable duties, according to Kant.

That the duty of self-preservation is a non-enforceable duty of virtue might appear to weaken the Kantian case against the legal permissibility of assisted dying on the grounds that the state ought not to make law aimed at compelling individuals to fulfill a duty that in fact they cannot be compelled by others to fulfill. This inference is mistaken, however. For even if the state could not compel individuals to fulfill their duty of self-preservation by outlawing assisted dying, the law could nevertheless shape attitudes toward assisted dying and hence influence whether the duty in question is fulfilled. Those inclined to shorten their lives encounter fewer obstacles if assisted dying is legally permissible. Indeed, a legal regime that permits assisted dying in effect offers inducements to violate our Kantian duty of self-preservation. The role of law here is thus asymmetrical: It cannot compel this duty's fulfillment, but it can certainly contribute to its non-fulfillment. Similarly, a person cannot compel a problem drinker to honor her self-regarding duty not to stupefy herself with intoxicating substances. Only the problem drinker can fulfill that duty. But a person can contribute to the duty's not being fulfilled by tempting the problem drinker with alcohol.

Kant Versus Kantians on Dignity and Assisted Dying

As discussed previously, supporters of assisted dying often appeal to dignity and associate it with recognizably Kantian values such as rational agency. Kant himself invokes dignity and claims that our rational agency grounds a duty of self-preservation that presumptively speaks against assisted dying. Here, I offer a sketch of why Kant's view appears to have the upper hand in this dispute.

Kant and supporters of assisted dying agree that because we are autonomous rational agents, we have broad rights to decide in what our welfare consists and how others may treat us. Our liberty to decide, independently of the wills of others, our own ways of life is a reflection of the special moral value of rational agency. Others are generally morally required to defer to our choices about our own welfare and way of life because we are rational agents, just as we are required to defer to theirs because they are rational agents. Our rational agency thus establishes broad moral permissions for agents to act as their own judgment concerning their welfare dictates.

For Kant, our rational agency serves a second moral role—namely grounding duties to respect our own rational agency—and in fact could not serve this other role unless it did so. Consider the first role, establishing a broad moral permission to choose our own ends and how best to pursue them. Suppose this discretion rested on some value or good V1 over which we had similar discretion such that V1 imposed no moral constraints on how we may respond to it. There would seem to need to be some still further value or good V2 that grounds our discretion over V1. If we had the same discretion over V2, then there would have to be some further value or good V3 that grounds our discretion over V2. But such a regress would have to terminate in some value or good of a different order or kind—a value or good over which we did not have this sort of discretion but which required our deference or respect. Kant believed that our rational agency is the value or good that halts this regress. Unless our rational agency imposed duties on us, including a duty of self-preservation, the discretion over own ends and the means thereunto that we enjoy would not be coherent.[12]

Hence, for Kantian supporters of death with dignity, our rational agency is purely a source of moral discretion or liberty. But for Kant, discretion cannot be the seed of morality. Discretion must ultimately flow from a value or good toward which we must defer. For Kant, there can only be something that counts as a person's good if persons are themselves sources of value. As David Velleman states,

> What's good for you wouldn't matter if you didn't matter. . . . What's good for a person is worth caring about only out of concern for the person, and hence only insofar as he is worth caring about. A person's good has only hypothetical or conditional value, which depends on the value of the person himself.[13]

Our rational agency thus does not merely confer value on our ends. It is also a value we must live up to or honor. A person's rational agency "isn't something that he can accept or decline, since it isn't a value *for* him; it's a value *in* him, which he can only violate or respect."[14] Our dignity (which, again, we possess due to our being rational agents) thus bars rather than authorizes ending our own lives and eliciting others' assistance in doing so.

I cannot claim to have offered a decisive basis for favoring Kant's understanding of dignity's demands over that of contemporary Kantian defenders of "death with dignity." Nevertheless, these remarks shift the argumentative burden onto assisted dying's ostensibly Kantian supporters to explain how the value of rational agency can both be the source of the moral discretion they embrace and also fall within the scope of that very discretion.

In summary, Kant's notion of dignity is distinctive in being universal, unified, equal, and unmerited. Only rational agency has dignity rather than

---

[12] J. David Velleman, "A Right of Self-Termination?", *Ethics* 109 (1999). 611–612.

[13] Velleman, "A Right of Self-Termination?", 611. See also Elizabeth Anderson, *Value in Ethics and Economics* (Cambridge, Mass.: Harvard University Press, 1993), 26.

[14] Velleman, "A Right of Self-Termination?", 625.

price, and we are therefore required to respect said agency by preserving the bodies through which we exercise such agency. Kant thus disagrees with contemporary Kantian defenders of a right to assisted dying about the role dignity has in the structure of our moral duties.

Exception 1: Permanent and Irreversible Cessation of Practical Agency

Kant's prohibition on suicide and assisted dying casts a wide net. Indeed, any prudential self-killing, in which one attempts to terminate one's life so as to result in a life perceived as happier, is seemingly ruled out. However, if there are conditions that result in individuals lacking the properties needed to ground dignity, then self-killing would not be wrong on Kantian grounds.[15] There are two kinds of "hopeless" situation wherein, I contend, Kant's prohibition would not apply precisely because such conditions are not met.

The first is relatively straightforward: The dignity we have due to our being practically rational agents is the basis for Kant's opposition to assisted dying. However, some individuals undergo conditions in which their practical agency has permanently and irreversibly ceased to function. Individuals in permanent vegetative states or those with severe dementia lack the capacities Kant associates with dignity, namely the capacity to identify ends worthy of pursuit and the means best suited to the realization of those ends. Such individuals, although biologically alive, are (from a Kantian perspective at least) practically dead, inasmuch as the properties that lend them their moral status are no longer present. In such cases, we cannot fail to respect that which provides human agents their dignity, for the properties needed for dignity are no longer in evidence. Thus, for such individuals to receive assistance in dying would not violate Kant's demand that we treat rational agents with dignity.

Granted, such situations are not commonplace, and such a conclusion obviously raises several practical issues, most notably, how to determine that a person has permanently and irreversibly lost the capacities associated with practically rational agency. Nevertheless, a recognizably Kantian position can allow that a person who, having been diagnosed with progressive dementia, wishes to receive assistance in dying once her

---

[15] Michael Cholbi, "A Kantian Defense of Prudential Suicide," *Journal of Moral Philosophy* 7, no. 4 (2010), 489–515, 493–494.

practical rationality has been wholly vitiated has a moral right to do so. In so doing, she is exercising a Kantian power to determine what will be done to her body once she lacks the capacity to exert power over it. She in effect directs others as to how her "practical remains" ought to be disposed of.

This conclusion should not be exaggerated. It does not entail that individuals who have permanently and irreversibly lost their capacities for practical agency are obligated to end their lives prematurely, nor does it carry the implication that others may end their lives. The absence of the morally relevant properties whose presence establishes a moral prohibition on self-killing does not entail a moral requirement of self-killing.[16] But those rational agents who assert a right to dispose of their bodies once their rational agency is no more do not act in opposition to the Kantian value of dignity.

Exception 2: Nihilism and the Lack of Categorical Desires

The second "hopeless" situation falling outside the Kantian prohibition on assisted dying occurs when individuals come to lack prudential reasons to continue living.

Many individuals undergo difficult stretches of life in which they are profoundly *pessimistic*. They may believe that they live in a world hostile to their ends, that they lack the skills needed to realize those ends, and that they have no legitimate place in the world and are burdensome to others.[17] For such individuals, happiness—understood in Kant's terms as the "complete well-being and satisfaction with one's condition" (G 4:393)—feels particularly elusive or remote. Unsurprisingly, pessimistic individuals may feel drawn to end their lives. The pain or frustration they feel at seemingly being unable to live a satisfactory or contented life may lead them to believe that a shorter life is better than one that continues forward.

Let us envision a more extreme version of the pessimist, the *nihilist*. The nihilist likely began as a pessimist, someone saddened by her apparent inability to realize the ends that constitute her happiness. But whereas the pessimist is still genuinely committed to particular ends, the nihilist has become wholly disenchanted, to the point at which she no longer has ends at all. Note that this is not to say that the nihilist has no wants. She may, for instance, have other-regarding preferences (e.g., desiring

---

[16] Michael Cholbi, "Kant on Euthanasia and the Duty to Die: Clearing the Air," *Journal of Medical Ethics* 41, no. 8 (2015): 607–610.

[17] Thomas Joiner, *Why People Die by Suicide* (Cambridge, Mass.: Harvard University Press, 2007).

that others she cares about flourish). She will also likely care about how her life goes so long as she is alive—that is, she will prefer not to suffer physical pain or deprivation. In terms made familiar by Bernard Williams, the nihilist retains *conditional* desires—desires predicated upon her continued existence. However, the nihilist is so disenchanted that she lacks altogether *categorical* desires—desires that give her a reason to continue to live.[18]

Both the pessimist and the nihilist have recognizably prudential reasons to seek to end their lives, but their reasons differ. The pessimist believes her life is (or will inevitably be) *bad*, an existence filled with pain or frustration at her ends going unmet. The nihilist, in contrast, believes her life is (or will inevitably be) *pointless*, an existence with no cognizable purpose or aim. However, Kant would likely argue that suicide or assisted dying would not be morally permissible in either case. In seeking to end their lives, both the pessimist and the nihilist run afoul of their duty of self-preservation and, specifically, fail to respect their rational agency as end in itself with dignity. Despondency, even out and out nihilism, does not appear to nullify the dignity we possess as practically rational agents.

I contend that although Kant's conclusions regarding pessimistic suicide are reasonable in light of his own moral doctrines, his conclusion that nihilistic suicide is similarly morally impermissible rests on a subtle error regarding rational agency, dignity, and their relation to price.

By Kant's lights, the nihilist is a moral agent. Despite her complete detachment from any ends whose fulfillment might constitute her happiness, she is nevertheless capable of moral reasoning, able to act from moral principles, and so on. In Kantian terms, the nihilist can acknowledge the force of categorical imperatives but recognizes the rational force of no hypothetical imperatives. The nihilist retains the dignity associated with moral personality despite having lost the dignity associated with humanity or practical agency.[19] For Kant, the absence of the latter dimension of dignity does not change the individual's status as an object of moral duties; she is still subject to all the same self-regarding duties as before, including the moral prohibition on self-killing.

Yet the nihilist is not a full-blown Kantian agent. For if she has permanently lost the ability to set ends (i.e., to identify states of affairs whose

---

[18] Bernard Williams, "The Makropulos Case: Reflections on the Tedium of Immortality," in *Problems of the Self* (Cambridge: Cambridge University Press, 1973): 82–100.
[19] Cholbi, "A Kantian Defense of Prudential Suicide," 502–503; Allen Wood, *Kantian Ethics* (Cambridge: Cambridge University Press, 2007), 94.

realization she is committed to and which she is thereby motivated to pursue), she has lost one of the two capacities that constitute her practical agency and dignity. This opens, I propose, a narrow alley for a form of suicide or assisted dying that falls outside Kant's prohibition.

To understand this, contrast the nihilist's prospective suicide with that of the pessimist. What Kant objects to in the suicide of the pessimist is her prioritizing her personal discretionary ends, whose worth is conditional on her setting these as her ends, over the unconditional worth of her own rational agency. The wrong in question consists in a transaction wherein the pessimist trades what has dignity (her own rational agency) for what has price (her happiness, or the ends that constitute it). But this analysis does not, indeed cannot, apply to the nihilist's suicide. Assuming that the nihilist is not engaging in altruistic suicide, ending her life so as to advance the ends of others, her personal reasons for suicide are not that a shorter life will be a happier or better life in any standard sense. Rather, her suicide is justified by appeal to the thought that continued existence has no point, not that it would have a point that will go unfulfilled. The nihilist is therefore not engaged in the transaction that, by Kant's lights, makes the pessimist's suicide morally impermissible. The nihilist is not trading her dignity for what has price. She is instead opting to jettison a future that has no value to her.

This conclusion is further vindicated by considering the previously presented regress argument used to defend Kant's conception of dignity . That argument held (roughly) that only if our rational agency has the priceless value of dignity are we morally entitled to authority over the priceable ends whose pursuit constitutes our happiness. But note that a nihilistic individual has no such ends over which to exercise her authority. Hence, this regress argument cannot get off the ground in her case, and so we cannot infer that her rational agency has the incomparable worth that (according to Kant) morally disallows her destroying the body through which that agency would otherwise be exercised. Stated more directly in terms of dignity, merely possessing the dignity of personality is insufficient to ground the Kantian prohibition on suicide and assisted dying. One must also have the dignity of humanity in order to be in a position to perform the morally objectionable transaction Kant saw as the root of suicide's wrongfulness. For absent the capacity to set ends that serve as categorical desires, we are moral subjects but not moral objects—that is, not beings whom we and others owe respect.[20] Nihilistic suicide thus cannot fail to respect one's

---

[20] Cholbi, "A Kantian Defense of Prudential Suicide," 507–509.

humanity or honor one's dignity. Kant erred, I propose, in holding that possessing even a fragmentary form of practical rational agency confers upon us a priceless dignity that bars suicide. The Kantian wrong of suicide is not best described in terms of its failing to respect human dignity. It consists instead of failing to respect human dignity by prioritizing the priceable good of one's happiness above what has dignity. That, I have argued, nihilists do not and cannot do.[21]

Admittedly, permanent or irreversible nihilism (like the permanent loss of practical agency considered in previously) is not a common condition. However, the sort of hopelessness and disenchantment I have ascribed to nihilism are not uncommon in those with suicidal ideation.[22] And so in what we might think of as the worst or most hopeless cases, those in which individuals either have lost the capacity for practical agency altogether or are irrevocably unable to identify ends they deem worthy of pursuit, suicide and assisted dying do not treat our rational agency (or our dignity) merely as a means. My modified Kantian view can thus embrace the moral permissibility of suicide in a handful of cases.

Conclusion

There are two kinds of "hopeless" cases in which, Kant's appeal to the priceless value of human dignity notwithstanding, the Kantian moral prohibition on suicide and, by extension, a prohibition on assisted dying do not apply. Note that neither case questions the fundamental soundness of Kant's arguments or overall moral stance. Rather, they illustrate that the scope of Kant's arguments is not quite as wide as he supposed because the psychological conditions presupposed in his arguments do not always obtain. For those with permanent and irreversible loss of practical agency and those with hopeless nihilism do not meet the psychological background conditions regarding rational agency that Kant's argument presupposes. Of course, even with these exceptions, the modified Kantian position on assisted dying I have articulated here establishes a much

---

[21] For a more detailed exposition of this argument concerning the permissibility of nihilistic suicide, see Cholbi, "A Kantian Defense of Prudential Suicide," 504–510.

[22] Martin Seligman has proposed that suicidal thinking accompanies learned helplessness. See Martin Seligman, *Helplessness: On Depression, Development, and Death* (New York: Freeman, 1992). Hopelessness also appears to be an indicator of suicidal thinking,. See E. David Klonsky et al., "Hopelessness as a Predictor of Attempted Suicide among First Admission Patients with Psychosis: A 10-Year Cohort Study," *Suicide and Life-Threatening Behavior* 41, no. 1 (2012): 1–10.

narrower moral permission than most contemporary liberal Kantian advocates of assisted dying would likely prefer. For if this modified Kantian position is plausible, then although death *with* dignity remains incoherent in Kant's eyes, some instances of assisted dying at least count as deaths *not at odds* with dignity.

SECTION 5 | Dignity and the Value of Life

CHAPTER 10 | Two Competing Conceptions
of Human Dignity

LUKE GORMALLY

THIS CHAPTER'S DISCUSSION of two conceptions of human dignity is concerned with the question whether one or the other serves to show either that the legalization of assisted suicide[1] is justifiable or that it cannot be justified.[2] It is important to keep in mind that the justifiability of *legalization* is the central issue. Assistance in suicide clearly involves an interpersonal relationship, and interpersonal relationships should be governed by basic norms of justice—norms which are rationally prior to rules of law and which provide criteria for assessing such laws as justified or unjustified. The law regulating any such relationship, as, for example, that between doctor and patient, should be consistent with those basic norms, which take the form of moral ("human" or "natural") obligations and rights.

In turn, claims about such moral or human rights are often defended as founded upon truths about the dignity of human beings. If the claim to be considered is that there is a right to assistance in suicide which the law should accommodate, the question arises whether there is a defensible conception of human dignity which underpins that claim. That is the question which the following discussion of two conceptions of human dignity seeks to answer.

---

[1] The phrase "assisted death" is somewhat ambiguous. One can assist a person while he or she is dying without that assistance being directed to bringing about that person's death. The unambiguous topic is "assisting (assistance) in suicide" because it is the act of assisting (giving assistance) rather than the condition of being assisted (or even the requesting that one be assisted) that is the object of the law's characteristic prohibition. When I use the phrase "assisted suicide" as the more usual locution, I understand it as equivalent to "assisting in suicide."

[2] The following text is a revised version of the paper I presented at the Zurich meeting in February 2014.

The first section is devoted to accurately characterizing assisted suicide. The second section reviews an autonomy-based understanding of human dignity which it is often claimed justifies the legalization of assistance in suicide. The third section explains and defends a conception of intrinsic human dignity as possessed by all human beings in virtue of their human nature. The fourth section briefly explains the anthropologies which underlie the competing conceptions of human dignity, finding the dualist anthropology characteristic of autonomy-based conceptions of human dignity defective and the anthropology which goes with the concept of intrinsic human dignity defensible. The fifth section argues that the egalitarian conception of intrinsic human dignity stands opposed to the legalization of assisted suicide and that the autonomy-based conception can provide no non-arbitrary basis for governing just relationships between doctors and patients. The sixth section explains the importance of the intention/foresight distinction for coherent restraints on doctors killing patients or assisting in patients killing themselves. The final section offers a summary conclusion.

I take the notion of dignity to signify the goodness a life possesses for what it is in itself.[3] This may also be referred to as the "worth" of a life.

What Is Assisted Suicide?

There is assisted suicide in the medical context *either* when a patient takes lethal drugs with the intention of causing his own death, the drugs cause his or her death, and the drugs are supplied at the request of the patient by a physician precisely with a view to bringing about the patient's death[4] *or* when a physician withdraws clinically assisted nutrition and hydration at a patient's request, the withdrawal is the cause of the patient dying when he or she does, and when the request is made precisely with a view to ending the patient's life and the physician does it with that purpose in mind.

Withdrawal of nutrition and hydration, when suicidally motivated, should not be excluded by stipulative definition from what counts as assistance in suicide. Clinically assisted nutrition and hydration is not *medical*

---

[3] See Aquinas: "'Dignity' signifies something's goodness for its own sake [*propter seipsum*]." III *Sent.* d.35 q.1 a.4 sol.1c. Quoted in John Finnis, *Aquinas: Moral, Political and Legal Theory* (Oxford: Oxford University Press, 1998), 179, fn. 219. And see note 24.

[4] The first part of this definition is close to that of L. W. Sumner. See L. W. Sumner, *Assisted Death: A Study in Law and Ethics* (New York: Oxford University Press, 2011), 18–19.

treatment—that is, it does not serve the distinctive goals of medicine.[5] A physician is obliged to withdraw medical treatments at the request of a competent patient. But physicians may reasonably refuse to be complicit in the withdrawal of the basic necessities of life when they know that the patient's demand for their withdrawal is motivated by the purpose of ending his or her life.

What is of critical importance in this understanding of assisted suicide is (1) the *intention/purpose* of the primary agent, the patient, to bring about his or her own death; and (2) the *sharing in that intention* by the secondary, assisting agent, the physician. For a secondary agent to share in a primary agent's intention is to act precisely with a view to achieving the primary agent's purpose. And one acts with a view to achieving the primary agent's purpose when one acts for the reasons the primary agent has for acting.

In general terms, the reason that motivates suicide is the patient's judgment that his or her *life is no longer worth living*, either because of intractable suffering, depression, the felt indignity of dependence, or a sense of "taedium vitae." The decision to assist suicide requires concurrence on the part of the assisting agent with the patient's judgment. Physicians are not mere technicians obliged to implement just any demand of patients but are obliged to act for what they reasonably judge to be of benefit to the patient. Normally the kind of benefit for which a physician is responsible is therapeutic or palliative. The case for a physician assisting a patient's suicide requires some extension of the notion of benefit to encompass termination of a life, and what purports to ground termination as beneficial is precisely the judgment that the life in question is no longer worth living. So a physician will think he has reason to assist in securing that benefit just insofar as he shares the patient's estimate of the worth of his continuing existence. In sharing the patient's reason for suicide, the physician shares the patient's intention.

So what is to count as the *worth, goodness, or dignity* of a patient's life is at the heart of the debate about legalizing assistance in suicide—*about whether there is a right to such assistance which the law should recognize.* It is for that reason that the concept of dignity is relevant. On one account, the distinctive status that dignity signifies derives from the exercisable

---

[5] Here I disagree with Sumner, *Assisted Death*, pp. 39–40. On the ends of medicine, see Luke Gormally, "The Good of Health and the Ends of Medicine," in *Natural Moral Law in Contemporary Society*, ed. Holger Zaborowski (Washington, D.C.: Catholic University of America Press, 2010), 264–284.

ability to confer meaning on one's life and so to determine its *worth*; on the other account, the worth of a human life derives from an understanding of human nature more comprehensive than that which focuses on the capacity for self-determination.

Dignity as Constituted by the Exercise of Autonomy

I shall largely confine myself to a brief exposition of a particularly sophisticated understanding of dignity as constituted by the exercise of autonomy,[6] that advanced by the late Ronald Dworkin in his book *Life's Dominion*.[7] Dworkin there makes a case for what he calls "precedent autonomy" with a view to establishing the authority of advance refusals of treatment, but the case has wider implications for the legalization of assistance in suicide and euthanasia.

Dworkin's understanding of the significance of autonomy is formulated in the light of a background distinction he makes between *biological life*, the life that consists simply in the biological endowment to which he seems to limit nature's contribution to our existence, and *the life of a person*, which has taken shape in virtue of that person's chosen commitments. For Dworkin, it is only the latter which possesses value. His low view of what he regards as "mere biological life" is fairly conveyed by his uninhibited references to patients who are irreversibly comatose as "unthinking yet scrupulously tended vegetables"[8] and, in the case of Nancy Cruzan, as "a manicured vegetable."[9]

He thinks that what has value in human life is the life of the *person* that has had value *conferred upon it* by the choices the person makes. Dworkin distinguishes two kinds of interest influencing choice: critical interests and experiential interests.[10] Each person's sense of whether their life is going

---

[6] This section draws heavily on my paper "Arguing from Autonomy and Dignity for the Legalization of Assistance in Suicide and Voluntary Euthanasia," *Acta Philosophica: Rivista Internazionale di Filosofia* 15, no. 2 (2006): 231–246.

[7] Ronald Dworkin, *Life's Dominion: An Argument about Abortion, Euthanasia, and Individual Freedom* (New York: Knopf, 1993). See Luke Gormally, ed., *Euthanasia, Clinical Practice and the Law* (London: The Linacre Centre, 1994), 120–126.

[8] Dworkin, *Life's Dominion*, 180.

[9] Dworkin, *Life's Dominion*, 192.

[10] Experiential interests are interests in the enjoyment of certain activities and experiences just for the pleasant experiences they are. The satisfying of experiential interests is not in general decisive for a person's sense that his or her life has gone well, unless one is what Dworkin calls a "critical hedonist"—someone for whom maximizing pleasure is the standard by which to judge a successful life.

well is governed by more or less self-conscious assumptions about what is worth achieving in life. Even if a person has not subjected these assumptions to critical reflection, they constitute a person's "critical interests"— the interests that determine a person's sense that he has made something of his life and not just wasted it.[11]

A person's critical interests, if he is reflective about the matter, are determined by decision, the kind of decision which underpins commitment, and it is commitment that determines the sort of consistency in a life which, in Dworkin's lexicon, is referred to as "integrity." Dworkin wants to qualify the idea that decision is foundational for integrity, and so for investing a life with value, by insisting that we remain exercised by the question whether we have got it right in settling on certain critical interests. However, that kind of question is to be answered, he says, by reminding

> ourselves of how it *feels* to believe that a given life is the right one. We feel this not as the discovery of a timeless formula, good for all times and places, but as a *direct response* to our own specific circumstances of place, culture and capacity.[12]

It is the consistent living up to one's commitments—integrity—which invests a life with value, the value Dworkin associates with the notion of human dignity. At the basis of those commitments is a radical exercise of autonomy in the choice of values. Hence Dworkin's fondness for the (in)famous "mystery" passage in the joint opinion of Justices O'Connor, Kennedy, and Souter in *Planned Parenthood v. Casey*: "At the heart of liberty is the right to define one's own concepts of existence, of meaning, of the universe, and of the mystery of human life."[13] Choices based on those conceptions, it is claimed, are "central to personal dignity and autonomy."[14] The notion that there are some basic common truths to be recognized in the shaping of one's life has disappeared to be replaced by a radical individualism difficult to distinguish from subjectivism.

The argument Dworkin advances is a sophisticated variant on an argument which is a commonplace in the bioethical literature that seeks to

---

[11] Dworkin, *Life's Dominion*, 201.

[12] Dworkin, *Life's Dominion*, 206, emphasis added.

[13] *Planned Parenthood of Southeastern Pa. v. Casey*, 505 U.S. 833 (1992), 851.

[14] Ibid. See the crucial role this text plays in the amicus brief to the Supreme Court in favor of legalizing assistance in suicide penned by Ronald Dworkin et al., "Assisted Suicide: The Philosophers' Brief," *New York Review of Books*, March 27, 1997: 41–47.

advocate the legalization both of assistance in suicide and of euthanasia. At bottom, L. W. Sumner's position is substantially the same. He treats "dignity" as an umbrella term precisely for autonomy and welfare/well-being considerations relevant to self-respect and loss of self-respect.[15] Autonomy is decisive because *"well-being is interpreted subjectively*, so that what is best for a person is ultimately determined by his own tastes, preferences and values."[16]

If the case for legalization is to be made in terms of benefit to the patient, it is a case which has to show what grounds there might be for judging that a patient no longer has a worthwhile life and would therefore be better off dead. Dworkin's contention that persons confer value on their lives through the shape they give them by the choices they make in the light of their critical interests is one way of articulating the widespread view that a person's exercise of autonomy (i.e., of the capacity for self-determination) lends unique authority to a person's valuation of his or her own life, for it is nothing other than their choices which has given to that life the value it has.

If it were true that the value of a person's life is uniquely determined by the choices that person makes, then, if he or she says that under certain conditions his or her life would not be worthwhile, that judgment may appear to provide sufficient justification for a physician either to assist in ending or directly ending that person's life. If a person's choices and a person's sense of his or her "integrity" (constituted by commitment to those choices) are uniquely determinative of the value of a person's life, then a physician can hardly have an alternative basis for disagreeing with a person's judgment that in certain circumstances the person's life would no longer be worthwhile.

Personal Dignity Constituted by Human Nature: Intrinsic Dignity

In contrast to the modern tendency to locate the origin of human value, and so dignity, in human willing, a more long-standing tradition locates it in human nature understood on basically Aristotelian lines—that is, human nature understood as informed by a principle of life which is goal directing: individual human beings are teleologically ordered to a range of objective goods constitutive of the fulfillment of their nature.

---

[15] See Chapter 4 of this volume.

[16] Sumner, *Assisted Death*, 34.

What shows the character of human nature in this respect is that our reasoning about how to live our lives, in answer to our interests in living well, finds fundamentally satisfactory answers about the worth of possible courses of action in a range of objective goods: life itself as something to be cherished, truth as knowledge of what really is the case and what ought to be the case (dispelling the ignorance that leaves us in the dark), justice as right relationships with our fellow human beings, friendship as communion of persons in shared loves of what is truly good, marriage as the faithful procreative friendship of a man and a woman ordered to the good of children, the enjoyment of beauty in what is glorious, and, not least, a right relationship to the transcendent origin of our existence. The existence of these goods strikes the reflective human being as goods for his or her own fulfillment; as a self-determining human being, one can and needs to have some share in these goods in order to flourish. The good that one possesses from the outset is the good of one's own existence. This, together with the freedom to share in the objective possibilities for flourishing, means that each of us matters, each of us exists for his or her own sake and not as a replaceable entity.[17] Although I can say "I matter," I have to recognize that every other human being matters on his or her own account because the goods constitutive of my flourishing are common goods, goods in which every other human being can in principle share in virtue of the nature we have in common. So, paradoxically, the unique worth, the dignity, of each human being is grounded in our common human nature and our capacity through choice to realize in our lives some share in the objective common goods perfective of that nature.

Intellect and will equip us for human fulfillment as capacities to know the truth and to choose to do what is good. We enjoy the freedom of self-determination to succeed or fail in these respects. So the radical capacity for self-determination is an intrinsic feature of our nature which makes for our dignity. But in its exercise, it does so not by some autonomous determination of what is to *count* as valuable but, rather, by our choosing to act in the knowledge of what are the true goods of the human form of life. And it is the necessities of preserving or realizing these goods that is the root of obligations. Because we are social animals, among these

---

[17] This is the proper foundation for the Kantian formula that we are "ends in ourselves." Modern conceptions of autonomy, pervasive in the bioethics literature, derive from the Kantian conception of human agency as rationally autonomous, meaning that it is judgments of practical reason that constitute what is to *count* as good—that is, the good is what I determine to be good. The authentic role of practical reason in respect of the human good is that of *recognizing* what is perfective of our nature as beings each fit to be an end in oneself.

goods is the fundamental good of justice, of right relationships between human beings.

Competing Anthropologies

The competing conceptions of human dignity reflect competing anthropologies. Let's consider first the anthropology which underpins the notion that dignity is constituted by that exercise of the capacity for self-determination which consists in the *choice* of what is to *count* as giving value, and therefore dignity, to one's life.

Characteristically, as we have seen, the anthropology involves a dualism between "biological life" and "personal life," the latter constituted by the exercise of autonomy. Personal life progressively supervenes on biological life and may progressively disappear, leaving biological life as a remnant without intrinsic value. Biological life, according to this anthropology, is of merely instrumental value in supporting the exercise of those psychological abilities in virtue of which people determine what is to be of value.[18]

This dualism is at odds both with our experience of the unitary character of our existence (of being always "organically living but only discontinuously conscious, and from time to time enquiring and judging, deliberating and choosing, communicating, etc."[19]) and with the manifest integration of sensory bodily activity and intellectual activity that occurs in the normal development of a human life,[20] an integration exhibited in the extraordinary range of human rational activities—in music, architecture, the domestic economy, the culinary arts, manual skills, the natural and social sciences, politics, games, philosophy, theology, the worship of the divine, and so much else. The capacities exhibited in these ways are ones which non-human animals simply cannot acquire. What accounts for the underlying unity of the organic, the sensory, and the intellectual?

---

[18] See, for example, Sumner, *Assisted Death*, 79.

[19] John Finnis, "Euthanasia and Justice," in *Human Rights and Common Good. Collected Essays of John Finnis: Volume III* (Oxford: Oxford University Press, 2011), 220.

[20] "The human being's mode of being an animal is specifically rational. Typically, his animal functions are modified or specified by rationality. Thus humans seek nourishment, shelter, sexual union, bearing and raising of children—all animal acts—in a specifically rational manner. Hence being rational, which enables one to have a first person perspective and allows one to view oneself from an objective standpoint, is, as Aristotle insisted, the specifically human manner of being an animal, that is, being an animal in a rational and self-conscious way"; Patrick Lee and Robert P George, *Body–Self Dualism in Contemporary Ethics and Politics* (New York: Cambridge University Press, 2007), 42. The entire volume is highly relevant to the present debate.

It cannot be the brain.[21] Why? Human beings respond to kinds as kinds, the intellect grasping intelligible structures in their material instantiations along with the characteristic activities of each kind. What are grasped are abstract concepts with general applicability, which enter into judgments and arguments. This capacity for abstract thought cannot in principle be reduced to or otherwise be entirely explained in terms of brain activity, even if brain activity is part of the story. For a thought to be material, it would have to be identifiable with something like a symbol or set of symbols encoded in the brain. But a concept could not be reduced to that kind of thing for an encoded symbol lacks the determinate content possessed by many concepts and the general applicability that derives from that fact, whereas an encoded symbol is indeterminate, being susceptible to varied interpretations.[22]

To illustrate: What concept would an encoded symbol of a triangle represent? "Triangularity"? "Trilaterality"? Depending on the symbol, neither the concepts of "triangularity" nor "trilaterality" may be the appropriate interpretation but instead the concepts of an "isosceles triangle" or a "scalene triangle." But in that case, what would represent "triangularity" or "trilaterality," which are distinct concepts even though it can be proved they co-instantiate? And what would differentiate the symbol for an isosceles triangle from that for an arrowhead?[23] The indeterminacy of the material cannot be the basis of conceptual thought, or the reasoning, judgment, and human willing in which concepts are exercised.

What makes possible the unity that gives rational directiveness to our lives is an organizing principle—a shaping *source* of activity—with a second-order capacity that is immaterial, shown in the immateriality of the acquired first-order intellectual abilities, through which we are *oriented to those human goods which fulfill our nature*. This organizing principle is what Aristotle called the human soul. It is because the soul (1) is the vital principle which gives unity throughout all stages of human development to the varied vital activities characteristic of human life—metabolic, sensitive, imaginative, intellectual, and volitional—and (2) does so in virtue of the radical (root) capacities inherent in the soul that any living human

---

[21] Sumner, for example, locates the capacity for intellectual consciousness in the cerebrum; Sumner, *Assisted Death*, 7.

[22] This line of reasoning is indebted to James Ross, *Thought and World: The Hidden Necessities* (Notre Dame, Ind.: University of Notre Dame Press, 2008), chap. 6, 115–127.

[23] I owe this example to Edward Feser. See further Edward Feser, "Kripke, Ross and the Immaterial Aspects of Thought," *American Catholic Philosophical Quarterly* 87, no.1 (2013), reprinted in Edward Feser, *Neo-Scholastic Essays* (South Bend, Ind.: St. Augustine's Press, 2015), 217–253. See also J. J. C. Smart and J. J. Haldane, *Atheism and Theism* (Oxford: Blackwell, 1996), 118–119.

being, however underdeveloped or debilitated, however afflicted by the "undignified" circumstances of dying, possesses intrinsic human dignity.[24] They possess the radical capacity which makes possible our sharing in the common goods constitutive of our flourishing in which our dignity is most clearly exhibited. First-order exercisable psychological abilities develop precisely in virtue of the radical second-order capacities inherent in the soul.

Implications for the Legalization of Assisted Suicide

I previously emphasized that the reasons people commonly invoke for wanting assistance in suicide at bottom amount to their judgment that their lives are no longer worth living. So in considering the justifiability of legalizing assistance in suicide, the question to be confronted is whether the law can reasonably accommodate judgments that a life is no longer worth living as an acceptable ground for assisting in the intentional causation of death. Are such judgments consistent with defensible claims about the nature of human dignity?

We may begin by asking whether, if a person judges that his or her life is no longer worth living, that judgment is compatible with respect for his or her intrinsic human dignity. And is acceptance by another—by a physician, for example—of a patient's judgment compatible with respect for the dignity of the patient? In agreeing with a patient who says, "It's simply not worth continuing to live in the wretched condition I'm in," is the physician thereby committed to saying that the patient lacks fundamental worth or dignity? Surely the judgments are distinguishable in what they refer to: in the one case, the worth or value of living in a certain condition, and in the

---

[24] See the fine statement by John Tasioulas: "The idea of human dignity is the idea of an intrinsically valuable status that merits our respect, a status grounded in the fact of being a human being. . . . Some important consequences follow from this understanding of human dignity. First, human dignity inheres in a human being from the moment of their coming into existence as an individual human being until their death . . . and this is so irrespective of the choices . . . or condition (e.g. embryonic, diseased, comatose) of the human being in question at any stage of their life. Second, since what matters is the possession of a human nature, the value of human dignity remains constant across different persons despite other ethically significant variations among them. A human being with impaired rational capacities shares in human dignity to the same extent as one with ordinary rational capacities. . . . Third, in the case of all human beings, their dignity confers on them a special value, and therefore justifies according them special consideration, as compared with all non-human animals. . . . Fourth, human dignity consists in an equality of basic moral status among human beings." John Tasioulas, "Human Dignity and the Foundations of Human Rights," in *Understanding Human Dignity. Proceedings of the British Academy 192*, ed. Christopher McCrudden (Oxford: Oxford University Press, 2013), 291–312, at 305–306.

other case, the value of a person. But if you talk about the value (or dignity) of a person, you are talking about something which holds good of the *actuality* of that person. To say that something has value although its *actual existence* lacks value hardly makes sense. There may be a notional distinction between the thought that a person's life is not worth going on with and the thought that the person, whose life it is, lacks value. But the former thought surely commits one to the latter thought. To think otherwise seems to rest on the assumption that the *being* of a human person is distinct from his or her ongoing life. But a human person just is a living human body, and the life of that person is the life of that body. Hence, to say that the ongoing life of a particular human being is not worthwhile is to deny value to the person whose life it is.

Human dignity understood as belonging to our human nature has a fundamental significance for our understanding of justice. As Elizabeth Anscombe remarked, "There is just one impregnable equality of all human beings. It lies in the value and dignity of being a human being."[25] It is this equality in dignity which is foundational for the claim that *every* human being enjoys basic human rights. A denial of this foundation is corrosive of this claim.[26]

Those who deny the existence of intrinsic human dignity and view dignity in voluntaristic terms—that is, as determined by a person's own choices—are mistaken for two reasons. First, their position is parasitic on an erroneous anthropology. Second, they face a fundamental difficulty over making their conception of how the value of a human life is determined compatible with a defensible conception of justice in the matter of killing or assistance in killing. As noted previously, it is common in the contemporary literature of bioethics to associate the notion of dignity with the exercise of personal autonomy in determining what is to count as the value of a person's life. But self-conferral of value assumes a developed capacity to do so, and there are developmental stages in the life of a human being during which no such exercisable capacity exists, and there can be periods of decline and debility during which such capacity

---

[25] See G. E. M. Anscombe, "The Dignity of the Human Being," in *Human Life, Action and Ethics: Essays by G. E. M. Anscombe*, ed. Mary Geach and Luke Gormally (Charlottesville, Va.: Imprint Academic, 2005), 67.

[26] See the observation of Robert Spaemann: "The dignity of a human person is violated in those cases in which it is stated implicitly or explicitly that this person does not count. Thus the Kantian formula of the 'end-in-itself' can be restated in a simplified manner: *everyone counts*." Robert Spaemann, *Love and the Dignity of Human Life* (Grand Rapids, Mich.: Eerdmans, 2012), 44. Note that for Spaemann, every living human being is a human person.

may be lost. At what point in development the capacity for self-valuation emerges and at what point it is lost are things unavoidably determined—and determinable—only in a more or less arbitrary manner. Because arbitrariness in determining something so fundamental as the value or dignity of a human life, and who therefore counts as a subject of justice, cannot be the basis for a just relationship between doctor and patient (arbitrariness being manifestly inconsistent with justice), one has to look to a sounder conception of human dignity—a conception both sounder in its own right and more fit to govern what rights in law patients and doctors may enjoy.

It is the concept of intrinsic human dignity which is foundational for our understanding of justice. That being so, the law cannot accommodate actions—assistance in suicide or euthanasia—the rationale for which is a judgment (that X's life is no longer worth living) which is incompatible with recognition of intrinsic human dignity. When we are discussing the legalization of assistance in suicide, we need to keep firmly in focus what kind of justification the law can accommodate for aiding and abetting killing. A patient's judgment that his or her life is no longer worth living overlooks or denies the intrinsic dignity or goodness of the patients' life, a dignity which stands in the way of treating that life as disposable.

Intention and Foresight

In the opening section, I emphasized the importance of *intention* in defining suicide and assistance in suicide, so I add some brief observations here on the moral significance of the distinction between intending an outcome and foreseeing but not intending it. It is a commonplace among consequentialist writers to collapse the distinction and to argue, in relation to the current topic, that a physician who administers opiates and sedatives to relieve otherwise intractable pain, foreseeing that they may hasten death, lacks compelling reasons not to aim at ending a patient's life because he has shown himself willing to act in a way that may or will cause death.

There are two good reasons for holding the distinction between intention and foresight to be morally significant. The first is that if foresight is regarded as equivalent to intention, then I will, for example, be regarded as just as responsible for killing men, as if it were my purpose to do so, if, for example, I build a fleet of fishing vessels or Formula 1 racing cars, for some men will foreseeably be caused to die, either by drowning or in crashes on the circuit. Hardly anyone will think it reasonable to say, "Never do any action from which foreseeably some death will follow." But if intention is on a par with foresight, people will also not think it reasonable to say, "Never commit the intentional action of killing an innocent man."[27] So there will be no such thing as an absolute right not to be murdered. The distinction between intention and foresight serves to hold in place the absolute character of those basic human rights which restrain conduct for the sake of just relations between human beings.[28]

The second reason is that what a person intends engages his will in a way that it is not engaged by what he foresees and permits to occur; insofar as he engages in the relevant intentional action he is committed to bringing it about, whereas no purpose of his is defeated if what he foresees as likely to occur fails to occur. But the commitment entailed by intention is not just that such-and-such a state of affairs should come about but that—precisely to bring it about—he or she, the agent, should behave in such-and-such a manner. Intentional action is self-defining action; it shapes character.[29]

Both of these reasons for holding the distinction between intention and foresight to be morally significant have a clear bearing on medical practice. Where physicians have been persuaded by consequentialist reasoning to think that there is no difference between intentionally causing death and foreseeably causing death, restraints on killing patients or assisting patients to kill themselves have been progressively relaxed, with increasingly wider categories of patients deemed eligible for being so "treated." And this is not just a grave injustice to patients but also seriously corrupting of the practitioners themselves.

Conclusion

We began with the question whether there is a defensible conception of human dignity which is capable of grounding a right to assistance in

---

[27] Here I adopt (and adapt) the wording of a text of Elizabeth Anscombe published in my paper "On Killing Human Beings" in Luke Gormally, David Albert Jones, and Roger Teichmann, eds., *The Moral Philosophy of Elizabeth Anscombe* (Exeter, UK: Imprint Academic, 2016), 133–153, at 137.

[28] See the powerful statement of the *Report of the House of Lords Select Committee on Medical Ethics* (HL Paper 21-1 of 1993–94; London: HMSO, 1994) at paragraph 237: "Society's prohibition of intentional killing . . . is the cornerstone of law and social relationships. It protects each one of us impartially, embodying the belief that all are equal. We do not wish that protection to be diminished and we therefore recommend that there should be no change to the law to permit euthanasia."

[29] See Anselm W. Müller, "Radical Subjectivity: Morality Versus Utilitarianism," *Ratio* 19 (1977): 115–132. See Solzhenitsyn's statement in his Nobel Prize lecture: "There is one simple step a courageous man can take—not to take part in the lie, not to give his support to false actions. Let this principle [viz. the lie that masks the method of violence] enter the world and even dominate the world—*but not through me*." Quoted by John Finnis, *Fundamentals of Ethics* (Oxford: Clarendon, 1983), 117. Finnis develops Müller's argument at 112–120.

suicide that should be recognized in law. The autonomy-based conception of human dignity which is widespread in the bioethics literature should be rejected. To make human worth or dignity dependent on a human being already enjoying exercisable capacities to determine what is to count as his or her worth is to adopt an arbitrary way of determining the kind of human worth that would warrant respect for basic rights and establish one as a subject of justice. Arbitrariness in the determination of who counts as a subject of justice is clearly incompatible with justice. The autonomy-based conception of human dignity can ground neither a supposed "liberty right" to assistance in suicide nor a "claim right" and should not govern doctors' dealings with their patients. Instead, doctors should rely on an entirely defensible egalitarian conception of intrinsic dignity. This conception means that there could not be a "liberty right" which would allow doctors to assist in suicide because they could not act on that false valuation of the life of their patient implicit in the request for suicide. Their obligation not to assist in suicide is not defeasible by their patient's request. Still less could there be a "claim right" to be assisted in suicide. The legal prohibition of assistance in suicide is one which both protects patients and preserves the integrity of doctors as healers and servants of life.[30]

---

[30] I am grateful to John Finnis, John Keown, and Christopher Kaczor for very helpful suggestions and comments on the penultimate draft of this chapter. The usual disclaimer applies, particularly because I did not follow all the advice given to me.

CHAPTER 11 | The Value of Life and
the Dignity of Persons

WILLIAM J. FITZPATRICK

ETHICAL DISCOURSE ABOUT end-of-life issues tends to be framed both in terms of the value or "sanctity" of human life and in terms of the importance of human dignity. These notions raise a variety of both interpretive and substantive questions, including how the two sets of issues interact. Talk of the dignity of human beings (or of persons or rational nature), for example, refers to a kind of *moral status* calling for certain forms of respect.[1] But the notion of dignity is also used in connection with an *ideal* for how a person's life should end, where a death with dignity is viewed as a goal to be promoted or perhaps even as something to which we have a moral right (supporting the case for a legal right).[2] What, then, does respect for *human dignity* require, and how does this relate to the ideal of a death *with dignity*? And how do both relate to claims about the value or sanctity of human life, especially in a secular and biologically informed context? Talk of the sanctity of life in fact invites questions not only about the intended notion of sanctity but also about what exactly it is that is being said to possess this value, which is often unclear.

Is what is sacred, as a literal reading suggests, the abstraction, *human life itself*—something that is manifested *in* all living human organisms? Human life in that sense is manifested not only in all of us but also in

---

[1] On human dignity as a moral status that might explain human rights, among other things, see Jeremy Waldron, "Is Dignity the Foundation of Human Rights?", in *Philosophical Foundations of Human Rights*, ed. Rowan Cruft, Matthew Liao, and Massimo Renzo (Oxford: Oxford University Press, 2015).

[2] This language is explicit in some physician-assisted dying laws, such as Oregon's "Death with Dignity Act," and in much ethical and legal discussion of end-of-life issues.

anencephalic infants (who lack the cerebral basis for consciousness), in patients in a persistent vegetative state (PVS), and even, apparently, in human beings who, despite having suffered whole brain death and thus been declared legally dead, have been kept on mechanical ventilation and continue to carry out integrative life activities.[3] Does the sanctity of human life imply that life is sacred even there, in a legally dead human being? Is human life sacred even as manifested in living human tissue cultures in a lab? Or should the focus be not on human life itself, in the abstract, but only on *the life of* this or that particular human organism, understood now as *the set of biological capacities and integrated activities constitutive of that organism's being alive*? If so, again, does this apply even where these capacities and activities are radically curtailed? Or, alternatively, perhaps life is not really the focus after all, despite the language being used, and talk of the sanctity of 'human life' is instead just another way of referring to the value of the concrete, living *human organism* itself, as when an individual is referred to as "*a* human life," meaning "a living human individual".

On this last interpretation, talk of sanctity of life overlaps with one sort of talk of human dignity, where both are intended to capture a special value or status of the human being and the importance of its continued existence. Other talk of human dignity, by contrast, focuses instead on a particular *capacity of* typical mature human beings, as in Kantian talk of the dignity (primarily) *of rational nature* as an end in itself. Still other appeals to dignity insist instead on a primary and irreducible focus on the *person* as the direct possessor of dignity, even where it is granted that a capacity such as rational nature is what makes the organism constitute a person in the first place. These differences will all affect our understanding of what respect for human dignity requires and how it relates to the value of life.

Adding to the complexity here is the fact that appeals to dignity are regularly made on both sides of debates over physician-assisted death (PAD).

---

[3] In a recent, well-known case, thirteen-year-old Jahi McMath suffered whole brain death (with a flat electroencephalogram and no intracranial blood flow) after massive blood loss and cardiac arrest due to post-surgical complications, and she was pronounced legally dead. Her family rejected the verdict and had her removed from the hospital and kept indefinitely (at a different facility in another state) on mechanical ventilation and a feeding tube. Although she is legally dead, the artificial support has maintained her body's integrated functioning. And this, according to Jeff McMahan's account, is sufficient to imply that her body is still technically *alive* despite the brain death (although he would not, of course, endorse keeping that life going under these circumstances). See Jeff McMahan, "An Alternative to Brain Death," *Journal of Law, Medicine and Ethics* 34, no. 1 (2006): 44–48. For a recent discussion of the ongoing McMath case, highlighting legal issues, see http://blogs.law.columbia.edu/publicrightsprivateconscience/2016/01/05/the-death-exemption-jahi-mcmath-the-right-to-life-after-death; accessed January 14, 2017.

Appeals to human dignity are often taken to join forces with talk of the sanctity of life to ground a strict moral prohibition against such practices. But other appeals to dignity are combined instead with an emphasis on respect for the autonomous choices of beings with dignity, where these choices often express a desire to die *with* dignity—that is, in a way that comports with a person's *sense* of dignity. These appeals are instead taken to provide moral justification in favor of such practices. Dignity can therefore seem to pull both ways.

My aim here is to impose some order on this perplexing mix of concepts and considerations, articulating and defending a plausible and morally attractive view. I argue first that the notion of human dignity is more fundamental than that of sanctity of life. Indeed, the idea of the sanctity of human life gets whatever legitimate meaning and normative significance it has only when viewed through the lens of human dignity, having no independent force. I go on to argue that human dignity is importantly person-focused and is best understood as that special form of value that is, in central cases, given appropriate recognition through an *irreducibly personal engagement that incorporates loving concern and respect for the person in question.* Finally, I take up complications involving so-called "marginal cases," which require a nuanced understanding of this person-centered focus and how it applies to particular cases.

The person-centered account contrasts sharply with views focused primarily on respecting the sanctity of the life manifested in a person or on respecting the value of some of her capacities, such as her rational nature, or the value of continued exercises of those capacities, or the value of the continuation of the human organism associated with her even against her wishes or even after she (as an embodied human subject) is gone.[4] Such approaches all misidentify the locus and nature of the ethical value at issue. On the proposed view, the reasonable wishes for PAD of a patient experiencing irremediable suffering and loss of a basic sense of meaning and value in continued life, for example, cannot be morally defeated

---

[4] I here follow McMahan in distinguishing between the human organism and the person, and I take him to have shown that we are *not identical* to human organisms. I do, however, hold that when the relevant sentient and/or rational capacities are present, the human organism *constitutes* an embodied human subject and/or person (although it ceases to do so when those capacities are absent), as discussed later. In that sense, I hold that although we are not identical to human organisms, which exist before we do and can exist after we cease (e.g., in a PVS), when we do exist, we are constituted by well-functioning human organisms with certain mental capacities. See Jeff McMahan, *The Ethics of Killing: Problems at the Margins of Life* (New York: Oxford University Press, 2002); Jeff McMahan, "Killing Embryos for Stem Cell Research," *Metaphilosophy* 38, no. 2–3 (2007): 170–189.

by appeals to the sanctity of life or by appeals to dignity that seek, in effect, to use her own life or dignity normatively against her. The notion of human dignity does have a role to play here, but it *supports* people making such decisions rather than throwing up moral obstacles to respecting their wishes.[5]

The Sanctity of Life: Biochemistry, Intrinsic Value, and Instrumental Value

Appeals to the sanctity of life address ethical issues that cannot be settled by biology. Still, such appeals must at least be consistent with what we know of biology, and one thing biology tells us is that life is a matter of natural biochemical processes, not quasi-mystical vital forces animating organic matter and operating according to special vitalistic principles. We can therefore set aside talk of sanctity of life in any sense that depends on vitalistic or other outmoded conceptions of life.

To be sure, biochemical processes have a wide variety of manifestations, some of which plausibly have special intrinsic value, as where they constitute sensation in sentient creatures and rational thought and agency in human beings. But there is no fundamental difference between comparable biochemical processes in human organisms and in non-human organisms, such as basic metabolic activities, that could give human life per se a special value or sanctity—as one might have thought if human life were permeated with or directed by a special human vital force or principle. So if basic metabolic activities, for example, have little or no *intrinsic* value in other creatures, then they cannot plausibly be thought to have significant intrinsic value in human beings either. The fact that they take place in the context of an organism with a genome that (due to often small genetic differences from those of other organisms) also normally leads to the manifestation of higher, intrinsically valuable biochemical processes such as rational thought does not mean that the basic supportive metabolic processes themselves have intrinsic value.

The primary value of such processes is instead *instrumental*, whether in humans or in other creatures, and it is here that they can naturally have a distinctive value in human beings by virtue of the special value of what they support. Metabolic activity in a human organism typically has special

---

[5] Practical concerns about the social effects of permissible legal policies involving PAD are a separate matter and are beyond the scope of this chapter. I am concerned only with moral issues in individual cases.

instrumental value by virtue of its sustaining in existence an intrinsically valuable human person and subserving intrinsically valuable person-involving life activities. There will be parallel instrumental roles in other creatures in connection with sustaining the existence of such organisms and subserving such higher-level life activities as are possible for them, but the particular instrumental role and value associated with subserving *persons* and *person-involving* life activities will not be shared by metabolic activity in other creatures. This can therefore make even basic human metabolic activity far more important than comparable activity in other animals.[6] But it is important that this difference in value is not a matter of some special *intrinsic* value adhering to *human life itself at all levels*; it is instead a matter of the instrumental relations human metabolic activities bear to specially valuable human persons and person-involving life activities, where "person" is understood (as it will be throughout) in the psychological sense of a rational agent, and person-involving activities are reason-involving activities characteristic of the lives of persons. More precisely, the previous claims about value provide a plausible model for the central case of human beings who presently constitute persons in the relevant sense. We take up atypical cases of human beings who are not "persons" in this sense in the last section.

What this suggests is that a primary theoretical focus on *human life* is a mistake. Although some manifestations of human life, such as person-involving life activities, have intrinsic value, basic metabolic activities do not, having instead instrumental value by subserving things that do have intrinsic value. The real question, then, is the following: Which things have the relevant intrinsic value, and what is entailed by respect for that value? And here we must be careful to avoid a natural mistake arising from a seemingly innocent slide from plausible thoughts about intrinsically valuable persons to a focus on human beings, understood as human organisms, leading to the thought that *this* is what has special intrinsic value and bestows sanctity on the life that subserves the continued existence of that organism. This might initially seem plausible for two reasons. First, in typical cases, the human organism, by virtue of possessing normal cognitive and emotional capacities, *also constitutes a person*, and we tend to focus

---

[6] This is not to deny that sentient non-human organisms and their activities also have some intrinsic value that needs to be respected in certain ways, perhaps grounding certain moral rights, or even constituting various forms of *animal dignity* grounding norms of interspecies justice, as Martha Nussbaum argues in *Frontiers of Justice: Disability, Nationality, and Species Membership* (Cambridge, Mass.: Belknap, 2007), chap. 6. My claim is just that the intrinsic values in play in these cases are less significant than those in connection with persons and their activities.

on such cases. Second, even where we recognize that the categories of *organism* and *person* can come apart (in atypical cases in which the human organism lacks person-constituting rational capacities), we also plausibly take the organism, which is, after all, still a human being, to retain some fundamental moral significance—often without diminishment. The effect is then to make it seem plausible to focus our theorizing about intrinsic value *directly* on the human being or organism and so then to see the sanctity of human life directly and generally in relation to its role in subserving the human organism as such. This is a mistake, however.

Even granting the point about the equal moral status of many human beings who lack rational capacity, it does not follow that the human organism is the appropriate general or direct focus for theoretical purposes of determining the source and structure of the values in play. Indeed, taking it to be so will be deeply misleading. I return in the final section to explore the ways in which in some cases human organisms that do not constitute persons in the relevant sense can *derivatively* take on the special dignity associated with persons, but that is a part of the story that emerges only after the primary account is developed. And the primary account cannot tenably focus directly on human organisms as such as the source of the special intrinsic value we are after, since again we have abandoned any human vitalism that could give the human organism *as such* some distinctive, elevated intrinsic value. Its special value, setting it apart from other organisms, must instead be understood by appeal to its special association with *personhood*, where it is personhood, or persons, or person-involving activities that are the source of special value or moral significance. In typical cases, the association is straightforward: The organism constitutes a person, and its life subserves personhood; in atypical cases, the association is less direct. The crucial point, however, is that the primary theoretical focus must be on what lies at the source of the special value in question, which is personhood or persons, rather than on the human organism as such, as if it were itself the source of a special value that could be understood independently of the larger story involving personhood. A proper theoretical focus will give us an accurate handle on human dignity, the value of life, and their implications.

Failure to heed this point has led to distorted thinking about the sanctity of life in both law and ethics. US Supreme Court opinions include defenses of the state's interests in "protecting human life" for its own sake, even where this is bad for the persons whose life it is.[7] Such thoughts about

---

[7] See McMahan (*The Ethics of Killing*, 465–466), who cites Ronald Dworkin's discussion of

the *unconditional* value of human life also underlie passionate and some-times bewildering calls for continued life support even in futile cases. One famous example involved the highly politicized fight over removal of a feeding tube from Terri Schiavo, who was in a long-term PVS resulting from extended oxygen deprivation that, according to all credible scientific evidence, had destroyed the capacity for conscious experience and left no prospect of regaining it, let alone anything approximating a life containing even minimal human goods. More recently and morbidly, the tragic case of Jahi McMath (see note 3) involved a fight with a hospital over removing mechanical ventilation from the body of a young patient who was legally deceased, following whole brain death, with no prospect of regaining more than metabolic functioning with mechanical ventilation and a feed-ing tube. Although part of the drive behind support for continued medical intervention was family members' denial and wishful thinking (e.g., the belief that as long as there is a heartbeat, there is a chance the patient will "wake up"), another major contributor, especially on the part of supporters citing the sanctity of life (often in a "pro-life" religious context), is pre-cisely the misplaced focus on the human organism and its continued life. Such a stance reflects not only a mislocation of value but also a failure to frame thinking about the value of human life within a proper acceptance of human mortality. It is a mistake to think that respect for life means that death is *always* to be fought, even when there is nothing to be gained but continued metabolic activity in a human organism irreversibly devoid of any human subject.

There is a better alternative. We should see the value of life neither in terms of any intrinsic value of metabolic activity in a human organism nor in terms of its instrumental value in keeping the organism in existence for its own sake but, rather (in the first instance), in terms of the instrumental value of subserving the intrinsically valuable person constituted by that well-functioning organism, and the higher-level activities of that person. That is, we should adopt a *person-centered approach* to the value of life rather than a metabolic or organismic-centered approach. To the extent that human life can be said to possess sanctity, it is only as contextualized in the previously discussed role in relation to persons (or in atypical cases, again, through the more complex relation described later). There is noth-ing about human life as such that has a plausible claim to sanctity when divorced from these relations and from acceptance of human mortality. It

Justices Rehnquist and Scalia, as well as the philosophical claim by John Finnis that human life has intrinsic value under any and all circumstances.

makes sense, then, in seeking to illuminate the structure of values in play here, to shift attention from the sanctity of life, or the associated dignity of the living human organism as such, to the dignity or intrinsic value of persons or personhood and person-involving activities.

Human Dignity, Rational Nature, and Persons

On a person-centered approach, human life has value primarily insofar as it subserves intrinsically valuable persons or personhood and person-involving activities. This means that the fundamental ethical issues in end-of-life contexts revolve around what is entailed by the respect called for by such intrinsic value. Our thinking about this form of value tends to incorporate the Kantian language of "dignity" and "ends-in-themselves."[8] This, however, masks an important divide between familiar intuitive thought about these things and the Kantian tradition.

When we speak of *dignity*, our focus is typically on the person herself as the primary subject of dignity, and talk of an end in itself is likewise a way of referring to the person as possessing a certain status—an inherent, unearned form of worth or standing—captured by talk of dignity and calling for distinctive forms of respect for the person. By contrast, although Kant and his followers sometimes speak this way as well, for them the application of such talk to persons is importantly derivative: What is primarily an end in itself, a subject of dignity, and an object of respect is "humanity," meaning the *rational nature in* persons. Talk of a person as an end then seems to be, as Thomas Hill puts it, "an abbreviation" for talk of rational nature as an end.[9] Indeed, in places Kant goes even further, saying that "the respect which we have for a person" is "really [respect] for the law, which [the person's] example holds before us."[10]

We thus have two importantly different ways of thinking about dignity, depending on whether the primary subject of dignity—and primary object of respect—is taken to be the *person* herself or instead a certain *aspect* of

---

[8] See Immanuel Kant, *Groundwork of the Metaphysics of Morals*, ed. Mary Gregor and Jens Timmerman (Cambridge: Cambridge University Press, 1998), 41–44 (Ak 4: 434–436), 36–38 (Ak 4: 428–429).

[9] Thomas Hill, "Humanity as an End in Itself," in *Dignity and Practical Reason in Kant's Moral Theory* (Ithaca, N.Y.: Cornell University Press, 1992), 38–57. Still, like other Kantian theorists, Hill does often speak of the dignity of persons. See Thomas Hill, *Respect, Pluralism, and Justice* (Oxford: Oxford University Press, 2000), chaps. 3 and 4.

[10] Immanuel Kant, *The Critique of Practical Reason*, trans. Lewis White Beck (New York: Macmillan, 1985), 81 (Ak 78). This echoes the claim in the *Groundwork* (14, Ak 4:401, note) that "the object of respect is . . . simply the *law*."

the person—that is, her rational nature (setting aside the further idea of the moral law as the primary object of respect). And this difference matters because respect for rational capacities *in* a person is not always equivalent to respecting *persons* as this is commonly and intuitively understood, and there are good reasons for preferring the latter and insisting on a non-derivative notion of the value or dignity of persons over a Kantian one.

Why, first of all, do Kantians hold that the primary focus of the dignity associated with personhood should be rational capacities rather than the person herself? The argument seems to go as follows. If persons possess such value and dignity, and merit such respect, this must be *because* of some special property they possess, which qualifies them as having this special status. And this property is plausibly rational nature. But if rational nature is what makes persons have their special status to begin with, then it must have that special status itself. Indeed, it will have that status non-derivatively, conferring such status derivatively on the person, and respecting persons must really just come down to respecting the rational nature in persons. As Allen Wood puts it, "Rational nature is precisely what makes you a person, so that respecting it in you is precisely what it means to respect you."[11]

We should, however, reject this inference. Even if we accept Wood's Kantian claim that "it is only because we are instantiations of this abstraction 'rational nature' that we deserve any respect at all," it does not follow that it is really rational nature that is the primary object of respect, and that respecting *us* just reduces to respecting *it in* us.[12] The possession of rational nature may instead transform the organism into a new creation—a *person*, which has a new significance as such and demands forms of respect that transcend respect for rational nature considered in itself. More generally, something can have special value by virtue of its possessing certain relevant properties without it being the case that those properties themselves are the primary possessors of that value, and we can cherish something in a way we would not have if it had lacked those properties without our cherishing thereby being directed primarily at those properties themselves or just reducing to treating those properties in certain ways. The properties can make their possessor an appropriate object of attitudes that take it now irreducibly as their target of concern.

---

[11] Allen Wood, *Kant's Ethical Thought* (Cambridge: Cambridge University Press, 1999), 144. See also Allen Wood, "Kant on Duties Regarding Nonrational Nature," *Proceedings of the Aristotelian Society Supplementary Volume* 72, no 1 (1998), 197–198.

[12] Wood, *Kant's Ethical Thought*, 144.

Consider the case of love, starting with romantic love. There are properties relevant to love for a spouse—properties such that, had the person lacked them, one might never have loved him or her as one does. It would be a mistake, however, to suppose that *what* one really loves is therefore primarily a laundry list of positive qualities in the person. Even if those qualities are important to one's loving the person, one's love for the whole living, breathing person does not reduce to love of the qualities, and the practical implications of love for the person are not reducible to anything about "furthering" those qualities in the person, although that may be part of it. This parallel is enough to suggest that Wood is moving too fast in taking respect for persons as rational beings to be reducible to respect for the rational nature in persons just because of the role played by rational nature in making the person an object of respect. It might be objected that the comparison to romantic love is limited by the fact that we might love one person and not another with many of the same qualities, whereas respect for persons does not work that way, being directed instead toward persons equally as possessors of rational nature. But we can make the same crucial point with the example of *agapeic* love, which is much closer in this regard to basic respect. Agapeic love for our fellow persons depends in typical cases on their having such properties as consciousness and various cognitive and emotional capacities, making them proper objects of such love (unlike our houseplants). Yet such love is not thereby a matter of loving those *qualities* in persons. Love remains a *personal stance and relation*, directed irreducibly toward the person as the object of that love, and there is no reason to suppose that what love of that person involves—the special sort of caring about her as an embodied, sentient, emotional, and rational being—can be exhaustively captured by anything about loving the person-making qualities she instantiates.[13]

This is highly suggestive for thought about *respect* for persons in response to their dignity, which is closely related to ideals of agapeic love, especially in the context of caring for patients. Just as love is irreducibly a way in which one relates to another *person* (or at least a human subject, in cases in which personhood is compromised, as discussed later) rather than to a *set of qualities in* the person, basic respect is plausibly also irreducibly a way in which one relates to persons rather than to a capacity in a person— even if that capacity is what inspires this sort of respect for the person.

---

[13] This point is even more compelling in the case of loving children, where it is even less plausible that such love is reducible to love for person-making qualities the child presently lacks but will one day have. This is similarly the case with basic respect for children (in connection with their present moral rights).

My respecting you as a rational being no more reduces to my respecting your rational capacities than my loving my wife as a smart, funny, kind person reduces to my loving intelligence, wit, and kindness in her (or our loving our fellow persons reduces to our loving the person-making capacities they instantiate). Because love is an interpersonal relation, the proper object of one's love is not a set of properties but, rather, the conscious subject of experience and agency who ideally might love one back. Similarly, if respect is an irreducibly interpersonal relation, then the proper object of respect—that which possesses the dignity that calls for such respect—is not a capacity, even as existing in a person, but rather *the conscious subject of experience and agency who ideally might respect one back.*

This alternative better captures intuitive thought about the dignity of persons and the proper focus of the respect such dignity calls for, which, like love, is essentially personal in nature. Indeed, the Kantian focus on rational nature or "humanity" as the primary subject of dignity and primary object of respect is distinctly implausible by comparison, even apart from applications to end-of-life contexts (considered in the next section). Rational nature consists in a set of capacities associated with practical rationality and possessed by all healthy, mature human beings.[14] At a minimum, this is taken to include the capacity to set ends through reason—to achieve reflective distance from our desires and impulses, to critically evaluate potential ends, and to judge some to be worth pursuing, thereby adopting them as one's purposes—and to pursue those ends through rational means.[15] Some commentators, such as Christine Korsgaard and Allen Wood, settle on this minimalist construal of the rational nature relevant to "humanity" and basic worth. But it is difficult to see why the *generic capacity to set ends* should itself be thought to have incomparable value and dignity, commanding our respect as the primary thing the moral law tells us is to be "cherished unconditionally." [16] Such elevated thoughts are fitting for persons, but they seem oddly misplaced when directed at a capacity.

This worry might be somewhat mitigated if, as Hill proposes, the capacity is expanded to include elements Kant later categorized under "personality," such as a capacity to recognize the moral standing of others or

[14] Richard Dean has challenged this reading of "humanity," taking it instead to refer to a good will, leading to a very different understanding of Kant's formula of humanity. See Richard Dean, *The Value of Humanity in Kant's Moral Theory* (Oxford: Oxford University Press, 2006). I explain why I am skeptical in William J. FitzPatrick, "Review of Richard Dean, *Value of Humanity in Kant's Moral Theory,*" *Mind* 116, no. 464 (2007): 1098–1104.

[15] Christine Korsgaard, "Kant's Formula of Humanity," in *Creating the Kingdom of Ends* (Cambridge: Cambridge University Press, 1996), 114, 124.

[16] Korsgaard, "Kant's Formula of Humanity," 111.

even the capacity to self-legislate moral principles and to follow them out of respect for the moral law.[17] Such a *capacity for morality* has a more plausible claim to incomparable value than the mere capacity to set one's goals. At the same time, however, focusing on the capacity for morality may then overly moralize the conception of what it means to respect an end in itself. As Wood points out in arguing for the more minimalistic construal, "Furthering rational nature [as an end in itself] requires furthering all the (morally permissible) ends it sets, not merely the ends it sets in response to duty," as we might suppose if we focused on respecting the capacity for morality.[18] More important, however, we have seen nothing in any case that forces us to focus on *any* capacity as the primary subject of dignity and object of respect, even granting the role such capacities play in transforming human organisms into persons who possess dignity and merit respect. Indeed, the comparison between respect and love strongly suggests instead a person-centered model for respect and dignity.

On this model, what is to be cherished unconditionally, as possessing absolute value and dignity, is fundamentally, irreducibly the *person*, and an account of what is involved in respect for a person should be guided by thought about what it is to respond appropriately to a person as such—not to a capacity possessed by a person but, rather, to *the whole person as a vulnerable living, sentient, cognitive, and emotional being*. For this, it is necessary to reflect on concrete human interactions, and thinking about end-of-life contexts will shed light on what is required by respect for persons in recognition of their dignity.

Dignity, Respect, and Sanctity of Life in End-of-Life Contexts

The contrast between the Kantian focus and the person-centered approach comes out clearly in cases in which a patient's losses and suffering have reached a point where she reasonably views death as a benefit rather than a harm, and she competently requests physician assistance in dying. The Kantian position can be seen most easily in the case of physician-assisted suicide. Kant's position is complicated by the fact that in *Groundwork* he does speak in person-oriented terms, although the claims he makes are unclear and puzzling. He says that suicide involves making "use of a

---

[17] Hill, *Respect, Pluralism, and Justice*, chaps. 3 and 4. Dean takes Hill to include a capacity for morality in the concept of humanity (*The Value of Humanity in Kant's Moral Theory*, 31).
[18] Wood, *Kant's Ethical Thought*, 120.

person merely as a means to maintain a tolerable condition up to the end of life"; in committing suicide, I improperly "dispose of a human being in my own person," which is morally problematic because "a human being . . . is not a thing . . . but must . . . always be regarded as an end in itself."[19] But although it is true that a person who commits suicide is using *her own destruction* as a means (in the ordinary sense) to her end of avoiding living in an intolerable condition, this does not imply that she is *making use* of *herself* as a *mere means* in Kant's sense. Indeed, it is difficult to see how she could possibly be doing so given that there is no coercion or deception and she is doing what she is doing for her own sake. (This is nothing like using a person as a mere means in Kant's case of a lying promise to get a loan, for example.) The same may be said about voluntary euthanasia from the doctor's point of view: It is far from clear that the doctor is treating the patient as a mere means, since again the doctor is acting for the patient's own sake, at the patient's request, using means that are neither coercive nor deceptive. So the claims in *Groundwork* are not much help here.[20]

Kant's position in *The Metaphysics of Morals*, however, is more clear. Suicide is there described as "disposing of oneself as a mere means to some discretionary end," and this is said to be morally problematic because it amounts to "debasing humanity in one's person."[21] This brings out the Kantian focus on the humanity or rational nature in the person and gives a clearer sense of what the Kantian worry might be. One's rational capacities, for Kant, are of absolute value and yet they are being destroyed for the sake of "mere inclination," making for a poor trade-off. Again, there are puzzles here that I mention only to set aside: How can suicide destroy one's rational capacities if those capacities belong to the timeless noumenal realm, as they must for Kant in order to manifest autonomy? Suicide destroys at most the temporal manifestations of one's rational capacities as given in experience, and it is hardly obvious why the value of a little more of *that* necessarily outweighs everything else, such as intense and humiliating suffering. But set that aside. Kant's main idea is that we are disrespecting the greater value of rational nature by making that trade-off. Indeed, Korsgaard notes that it is worse than that—not just a bad trade-off but also an incoherent one, because the merely "relative end" of avoiding suffering "must get its value from the thing that is being destroyed

[19] Kant, *Groundwork*, 37–38 (Ak 4:429).

[20] McMahan, *The Ethics of Killing*, 484.

[21] Immanuel Kant, *The Metaphysics of Morals*, trans. Mary Gregor (Cambridge: Cambridge University Press, 1991), 219 (Ak 423).

for its sake," namely rational nature.[22] Humanity or rational nature is the very *source* of the value of all relative ends, including the end of avoiding terrible and pointless suffering, and so it is doubly offensive to humanity to sacrifice it for one of those ends. David Velleman puts the point as follows: "The value of what's good for a person is only a shadow of the value inhering in the person."[23]

This line of reasoning has little attraction or plausibility, however, for anyone not already invested for other reasons in highly contentious theoretical claims associated (mostly) with Kantian constructivism.[24] There is no independent plausibility in the thought that the end of avoiding or escaping terrible and pointless suffering has no inherent value and derives any normative significance it has from rational nature as the source of *all* value and normativity. The absence of rational nature in non-human animals does not undermine the inherent disvalue or significance of their suffering (which would contribute to the badness of a state of affairs even in a world entirely devoid of rational agents), and although rational nature is present in typical cases of human suffering, reflection on the experience and impact of suffering on the whole human person makes it overwhelmingly plausible that it has evaluative and normative significance *in its own right*, independently of relations to or further impacts upon the exercise of our power of rational choice.

The experience of watching a loved one suffer and decline underscores this point. Suffering has a *direct and intrinsic negative impact* on a person's flourishing, given that a person is, in part, a sentient being. Such suffering, together with the loss of basic ability and control, including control of bodily functions and movement and psychological composure, also negatively impacts a person's flourishing by eroding her *sense* of dignity, the preservation of which is an important component of flourishing for persons. Part of *loving a person* is caring about her flourishing and recognizing that physical and emotional pain, decline, and erosion of a sense of dignity are inherent sources of disvalue and of reasons to mitigate such anguish.

Keeping this perspective in mind is revealing: It is difficult when engaged in this loving relation to another person to find much plausibility

---

[22] Korsgaard, "Kant's Formula of Humanity," 126.
[23] J. David Velleman, "A Right of Self-Termination?", *Ethics* 109, no. 3 (1999): 606–628, 613. For excellent critical discussion of Velleman's argument, which I cannot take up beyond the more general critique of such a position here, see McMahan, *The Ethics of Killing*, 473–485.
[24] For criticism, see William J. FitzPatrick, "The Practical Turn in Ethical Theory: Korsgaard's Constructivism, Realism, and the Nature of Normativity," *Ethics* 115, no. 4 (2005): 651–691.

in a theoretical stance that downplays the significance of a person's suffering and sense of dignity while deferring instead to the dignity of a subset of that person's capacities and suggesting that what is of overriding importance is a few more weeks of exercises of the person's choice-making power. Such a stance in fact makes the very type of mistake it accuses the defender of PAD of making: It gets the value priorities backwards, in this case glorifying one aspect of the person—rational capacity—as the primary object of value and dignity, while in fact this capacity has whatever value it has only *contextually* as *one aspect of the flourishing of the person to which it belongs.*[25] The person and her flourishing are what primarily matters—and this despite the fact that rational capacity is precisely what makes persons qualify as persons to begin with. The latter role is just a different issue from that of the primary focus of value, and the two should not be conflated: Rational nature makes a human organism constitute a person, but the locus of value is the person and her flourishing, not rational nature itself as something set apart from the rest of the person and other elements of her flourishing.[26]

Again, this fact comes into sharp focus when we consider persons from a perspective of loving concern, and my claim is that this is also how we should see things from the perspective of basic respect. Such respect is appropriately directed toward the person as a whole person, not simply toward an aspect of that person; as a response to the dignity of the person it will take seriously the person's overall flourishing, including the importance *to* the person of her own *sense* of dignity, respecting the judgments she makes about her life rather than focusing unwaveringly on the preservation and continued exercise of her choice-making capacities for their own sake. This is what it is to respect a person, and it precludes downplaying a terminal patient's anguished desire to be spared further suffering and humiliation as "mere inclination"; it precludes seeing such a desire as a merely "discretionary end" that owes its value entirely to the person's rational capacities and so loses out automatically to a few more weeks of miserable exercise of those capacities (assuming that they remain intact

---

[25] Cf. McMahan's objection that Velleman's view "treats the person, in effect, as a mere housing for his rational nature, or the medium in which the rational nature is manifest" (*The Ethics of Killing*, 479).

[26] Cf. McMahan, *The Ethics of Killing*, 479, 482–483. Recognizing this point is compatible with granting the Kantian claim that rational nature should not be used merely as a tool for the promotion of inclination, as with using one's reason simply to pursue hedonistic ends without concern for morality. The claim I am defending in this section is just that, *contra* the Kantian position, suicide or assisting someone in dying need not in any way amount to such a mistreatment of her rational nature or a violation of her (or of her dignity) as a person.

at that point). If it is the person herself who ultimately matters, then her welfare as a whole person—as an embodied rational being with an animal as well as a rational nature—will matter *directly* and *in its own right*. And that is what we should be responding to both in loving persons and in respecting them, even, if necessary, at the expense of the very properties that made them appropriate objects of such respect in the first place. Helping a person to die under such circumstances, out of concern for her welfare and respect for her autonomous wishes and for her own sense of dignity, is precisely *to respect the person*. There is simply no good reason to think that such assistance in dying somehow always and essentially disrespects the person in question.[27]

The same points apply to claims about the sanctity of life. I argued earlier that while some life activities have intrinsic value, as with higher-level activities normally constitutive of human flourishing, the value of basic metabolic functioning in human beings is instrumental insofar as it supports intrinsically valuable persons or personhood and higher life activities. I have now argued that the primary focus for such intrinsic value is on *persons*, with valuable *capacities* or *activities* always to be assessed contextually by considering their place in the flourishing of persons. It gets things fundamentally backwards to object to a patient's request for PAD by appealing to the dignity or incomparable value of her rational nature, as if this could require her to continue living in conditions she finds intolerable in order to maximize the exercise of rational abilities. In the same way, it gets things backwards to object to her request on grounds of the alleged sanctity of the life she reasonably judges to be more of a burden than a benefit to her. The instrumental role life plays in keeping a human organism going is normally of great value but not always, and where quality of life is so compromised that a person reasonably rejects it, there is no independent moral leverage in an appeal to the sanctity of her life that could plausibly override her judgment and choice of PAD. Moral authority in such matters lies with the person who is *the end for the sake of which life and rational capacities matter when they do*, rather than the other way around.

Marginal Cases and Species Membership

I have so far focused on cases in which personhood is realized due to the possession of rational capacities that make the human organism constitute

---

[27] As in much else, I am in agreement here with McMahan, *The Ethics of Killing*, 476 f.

a person, and I have spoken as if the special moral status we intend to capture with talk of dignity is always associated directly with such person-hood. Such a view, however, is an oversimplification, and something must now be said about "marginal cases" involving human beings who lack the relevant rational capacities. For it is certainly not my view that small children (who possess such capacities only potentially), the severely mentally handicapped (who do not possess even the potential for them), and those afflicted with dementia (who have irretrievably lost them) lack the basic human dignity I have ascribed to persons. But how can we understand their possession of this special moral status associated with rational nature if they individually lack those rational capacities?

It has become common to dismiss the suggestion that species member-ship could provide an answer here, whether through now familiar accu-sations of "speciesism" or more developed worries about complications involved in appeals to species.[28] This, I believe, is a mistake. The appeal to species membership, properly understood, just reflects the plausible idea that an entity's moral status is not simply a function of its "individual qual-ifications," such as its present cognitive or emotional capacities, but is sen-sitive to other considerations as well. That is, we should not think of moral status on the model of a candidate's status in an ideal job search, where *all* that is relevant are indeed the candidate's individual qualifications and there should be no discrimination based on racial or gender group mem-bership, for example. Instead, when thinking about the normative signif-icance of a living being, it is entirely plausible that in addition to taking account of its individual mental properties, we should also be sensitive to the *fundamental kind* of thing we are presented with.[29] It is a mistake to think that when facing a patient with dementia we must, out of a sense of egalitarian consistency or fairness to other animals, disregard the fact that this is a human being we are dealing with and focus only on his individual mental capacities, attributing to him only whatever status we are prepared to ascribe to healthy non-human animals with comparable properties. Although we should no doubt treat non-human animals far better than we do, and many have an inherent moral status as sentient creatures that plau-sibly grounds moral rights against certain treatment by moral agents, it is

---

[28] On "speciesism," see Tom Regan, *The Case for Animal Rights* (London: Routledge and Keegan Paul, 1983); and Peter Singer, *Practical Ethics*, 2nd ed. (Cambridge: Cambridge University Press, 1993). For complications on ethical appeals to species membership, see McMahan, *The Ethics of Killing*, 209–216.

[29] Cf. Thomas Scanlon, *What We Owe to Each Other* (Cambridge, Mass.: Harvard University Press, 1998), 185–186.

hardly beside the point when thinking about moral status to acknowledge that a human being suffering from dementia is metaphysically a very different kind of thing from a healthy pig, despite similarities in individual mental capacities.[30]

We should be appalled at the suggestion that due to this patient's diminished capacities it is now up for discussion whether he might be a candidate for medical experimentation or organ harvesting or painless extermination to save resources, on the grounds that his mental capacities are not inherently different from those of various non-human animals for which such things are at least a live issue. We could not, I think, claim to harbor a proper respect for persons while being prepared to take on such an attitude toward someone as soon as he is afflicted with major dementia or a brain injury—or similarly toward a small child who has not yet developed rational capacities or a severely handicapped child who never will. It matters in each case that we are confronted not only with a being with limited mental capacities but also with a being who is fundamentally a certain *kind* of thing: *a member of a "person-species"*—that is, a species whose normal mature members possess person-constituting rational capacities.

The claim is not that this condition is *necessary* for possessing the moral status associated with personhood: Jeff McMahan's hypothetical example of Superchimp—a genetically modified chimp who individually possesses rational capacity and so plausibly has the same status we enjoy, although he does not belong to any person-species—shows that individual possession of the relevant properties is sufficient by itself for special moral status, even without membership in a person-species.[31] Rather, the claim is that such membership is *likewise sufficient* for special moral status, as supported by reflection on small children, the severely handicapped,

---

[30] McMahan objects that it is unclear why, if we are not identical to human organisms, our species membership should determine the kind of thing we fundamentally are (*The Ethics of Killing*, 216). The answer is that although we are not *identical* to organisms, for the reasons he gives, we are nonetheless *constituted* by *organisms-instantiating-certain-capacities*—a claim that is compatible with our not existing at all times that our organism exists. And that is a sufficiently intimate relationship to support the species-membership claim about the kind of thing we fundamentally are.

[31] See McMahan, *The Ethics of Killing*, 211, 216. Note that my appeal to membership in a person-species is very different from Carl Cohen's in "The Case for the Use of Animals in Biomedical Research," *New England Journal of Medicine* 315, no. 14 (1986): 865–870. He takes such membership to be a necessary condition for the possession of any rights at all, whereas I grant that many non-human animals possess moral rights. My appeal to membership in a person-species is relevant only to elevating marginal members to the status of full dignity characteristic of the species, and it does not exclude non-members from having various kinds and degrees of moral rights (or even, in the case of Superchimp, full rights and dignity).

and those suffering from dementia, where a focus on individual properties alone misses something crucial. There is a certain dignity associated
with a person-species by virtue of the dignity attaching to the *persons
constituted by* its normal, mature members, and given the role of species
in determining fundamental kinds for living things, this dignity extends
generally to members of that species. The dignity associated with *Homo
sapiens*, as a person-species, thus extends to all human beings, regardless of whether they all individually possess the special mental charac-
teristics that make their kind a special one—although naturally the sort
of treatment demanded by such dignity will vary with the circumstances,
as discussed later. The same point applies to possible extraterrestrial
person-species: There is no "speciesist" favoring of *H. sapiens* over other
person-species.[32]

There are no doubt many difficulties to be addressed by such a view.
Attempts to settle the metaphysical issue of kind membership by appeal
to biology, for example, face various complications. This is not because
we are implausibly trying to extract normative significance directly from
biological facts, which we are not: The biology is only indirectly relevant, in helping to establish metaphysical facts about kinds, which latter
are plausibly relevant for the reasons given. Still, as McMahan notes, the
appeal to biology is itself complicated because neither genetic essential-
ism nor statistical genetic criteria are promising ways of capturing species
membership for such purposes, as brought out, for example, with spectrum arguments.[33] Some of these difficulties can be avoided by focusing
on a being's place within a relevant *lineage* rather than genetic statistics,
but it must be accepted that however we seek to understand the relevant
kinds, there will inevitably be gray areas (e.g., during species transitions)
and puzzle cases, especially when we introduce hypothetical technologi-
cal manipulations of a creature's properties that set it relevantly apart from
others in its lineage. We should just grant that there will be many cases in
which the application of the kind-oriented consideration will be unclear
or even untenable. Even so, it does not follow that it does no moral work
in straightforward cases involving those who are uncontroversially human

---

[32] Note that this claim has no direct implications for debates over abortion because the central
complication there is precisely over whether embryos or fetuses at various stages are actually
human beings in the relevant sense (full-fledged members of a person-species) or still only early
stages of human beings under construction. The proposed view does not imply that the latter
have the same moral status as actual human beings. In general, being *human* (as opposed to, e.g.,
bovine), which applies even to single somatic cells, obviously does not entail being *a human being*,
so it is important to avoid any easy slide from the former to the latter.

[33] McMahan, *The Ethics of Killing*, 212–217.

beings, born of other human beings, who lack typical human rational capacity whether through immaturity, congenital defect, injury, or disease. We need not be in a position to draw unambiguous conclusions about all cases, real or imagined, in order to recognize the human dignity that extends to individuals in these cases because of *what they are*, quite apart from *what they can individually do*.

What is morally entailed by such respect? In the extreme case, we may have a human being in a PVS, where there is no longer any subject present, and so, in the absence of any experience, no longer any interests that might be furthered or frustrated. Here, the dignity that attaches to the human being in the kind-oriented way has minimal implications, no longer speaking to the protection of interests.[34] It surely requires respectful handling, and plausibly grounds a prohibition against killing the organism without prior consent in an advance directive. But it is not clear that any residual dignity or past wishes are enough to ground any positive duty to continue to provide resources to keep the organism alive at this point. Surely there is no positive duty to keep a clinically dead human organism "alive" on mechanical ventilation (maintaining integrated functioning) following whole brain death, and there is no actual greater benefit in keeping a clinically living human organism in a PVS alive: The remaining life processes are not those that plausibly have intrinsic value, and in the absence of such value there is no longer the usual instrumental value of the metabolic activities either. Neither the derivative respect for human beings stemming from dignity-based respect for persons nor appeals to the usual value of human life entail a duty to keep the organism and its metabolic activities going under these circumstances, and still less could they plausibly be used to contravene the earlier wishes of the person once associated with that organism that its life not continue in such circumstances.

In less extreme cases, involving major dementia, for example, the human organism still functions in such a way as to constitute a *living, embodied human subject*, even if not a person in the strict sense of a rational agent, and an important range of interests are still obviously present. Here, despite the loss of personhood, there is still *someone* present to serve as the object of our continuing love. And the person-based dignity that still attaches to such a human being in the kind-oriented way makes her equally a proper object of respect—specifically respect for her as (1) a member

---

[34] The same point applies to the case of anencephalic infants, although the role played in a PVS case by the earlier person via an advance directive would instead have to be played by a proxy decision-maker.

of a person-species (2) who also constitutes an embodied human subject. Such respect, in recognition of the dignity that extends to her, entails the same special degree of concern with this human being's interests as with the interests of any paradigm person, even if her interests are naturally more restricted due to her diminished capacities. Indeed, it is precisely because of all this that it is so natural, and appropriate, to use the term "person" in a broader sense that applies to all such "marginal cases"—the sense in which it will seem perfectly obvious that the residents of neonatal intensive care units or of nursing homes are *persons* (what else?). But it is important to arrive at this use through the sort of account offered here, starting with the narrower sense of "person" and its significance, for the reasons given previously.

The person-centered approach I have defended is therefore compatible with extending to so-called "marginal cases" the same kind and degree of respect owed to persons (in the narrow sense) because personhood can ground the relevant dignity not only directly by being manifested in the individual case but also indirectly via kind-oriented considerations. Moreover, the latter move achieves this plausible level of egalitarianism without "lowering the bar" for which *individual* properties count as qualifying a being for the special moral status associated with human dignity, as Tom Regan does, which would result in a radical extension of this special, very high moral status to all animals that are "experiencing subjects of a life," making for a much less plausible egalitarianism.[35] The proposed view thus offers a moderate solution to the "problem of marginal cases," preserving plausible intuitions about the equal moral status of atypical human beings while remaining at bottom a person-centered view.

Previously, I argued that the person-centered account supports a person's reasonable choice to seek assistance in dying in a dignity-preserving way rather than allowing appeals to the value of her life or the dignity of her rational capacities to undermine such choices. The kind-oriented extension of dignity does not change this: The moral authority of a person's reasonable wishes in such cases, grounded directly in her primary dignity, cannot be overridden by appeal to the derivative dignity she possesses as a member of a person-species, as if the latter had an independent normative force that could somehow override the force of the dignity at its source, demanding continuation of a life the person herself finds intolerable. Such an application of the kind-oriented notion of dignity would

---

[35] Regan, *The Case for Animal Rights.*

be incoherent. And the same point applies to cases in which a person has written an advance directive refusing cardiopulmonary resuscitation or antibiotics for pneumonia in circumstances of advanced dementia: It would make no sense, on the proposed view, to appeal to the derivative, kind-oriented dignity of a human being in those circumstances to override the autonomous wishes of the actual person who was once constituted by that human being.

There are, of course, still complicated ethical issues to work out here. For example, although a person plausibly has the moral authority to expect the previously mentioned sort of advance directive to be carried out, it is far from clear that such moral authority would extend to an advance directive involving active euthanasia (assuming it were legal). Such a directive might be acceptable with respect to PVS, where one might request that one's organism's life be ended to enable organ donation at that point (again, assuming legality), because there are no competing interests on the part of the human being at the time in question. But in the case of dementia still involving a human subject of experience and associated interests, there are complications involving personal identity between the earlier person and the current patient, among other things, that cast doubt on the moral authority of the earlier person to call for the active termination of that later human being.[36] My present purpose has not been to suggest that end-of-life quandaries will always admit of straightforward solutions, but just to lay out and defend a framework for understanding human dignity and the value of life that keeps the person always at the focus of our ethical thinking.

---

[36] See Thomas Mappes, "Some Reflections on Advance Directives," *APA Newsletters: Newsletter on Philosophy and Medicine* Vol. 98, no. 1 (1998): 106–111.

SECTION 6 | Dignity and Rights

CHAPTER 12 | ## Could Suicide Really Be a Fundamental Human Right?
A Triple Threat

MARGARET P. BATTIN

THREE AND A HALF DECADES AGO, 1980 to be exact, when I was new
in the field of bioethics—itself then also new in the staid old discipline
of philosophy—I wrote a paper that tried to make a seemingly absurd
point.[1] Suicide, it argued, is a fundamental human right—not just something to be excused or understood in some cases, not just something permissible sometimes, not just an ordinary liberty right, but a *fundamental*
one. This seemingly outrageous claim was based in an account of human
dignity.

Now, so many years later, after decades of attention to the practical context of physician-assisted suicide, as I watch legal change in the
United States and Europe, as I see not only my friends and colleagues
take on the patina of age but also entire nations graying, as I listen to the
lifelong suffering of friends who have lost a child to suicide and heard
the terrifying stories of those who made serious, nearly lethal suicide
attempts but survived, and as I have lain next to the person I've loved
most in the world while, at his own request, his life-prolonging ventilator
was removed—now it is time for me to rethink this issue of dignity and
suicide. Suicide, a *fundamental* human right? Rooted in *dignity?* What
was I thinking?

---

[1] Margaret Pabst Battin, "Suicide: A *Fundamental* Human Right?", in *The Least Worst Death*
(New York: Oxford University Press, 1994), 277–288.

Suicide as a Right?

The case that suicide is a fundamental human right, or any sort of right for that matter, might seem to flounder immediately when confronted with the sad parade of suicides that actually occur, logged at almost 40,000 a year in the United States alone, and nearly a million subfatal attempts, each a fraction of an enormous global toll. Some are star-crossed lovers, some are workers or farmers or high-flying financiers caught in unbearable financial stress, some are users of physically or mentally devastating drugs, and many, many are caught in the vise-like grip of depression.

So how could suicide conceivably be a *fundamental* right?

Rights, of course, come in a variety of forms: liberty rights, claim rights, legal rights, constitutional rights, derivative rights, and so on, and of course the fundamental rights that are typically iterated in manifestoes of various sorts—life, liberty, fraternity, freedom from want, the pursuit of happiness, and so on. Rights are of differing scope and have different limitations, but a right to *suicide* may seem to be none of these, and especially not one of the sorts of fundamental rights traditionally listed in the various celebrated manifestoes.

Of course, that suicide is not included in any compendium of rights could depend on the negative, pejorative connotations of the term "suicide" itself—among them, the connotations of *sin*, associated with theologies from medieval Catholic thought to American Protestantism; of *cowardice* and *crime*, asserted by thinkers from Aristotle to Blackstone and on; and of *mental illness* or psychopathology, articulated by Esquirol and Freud.[2] Subtract out these negative connotations and call this action *self-initiated death*, and call the medical practice that is the focus of such volatile political discussion not *physician-assisted suicide* (as detractors label it) but, rather, *physician-aided dying.* Does this change the way we might think about "suicide," or rather "self-initiated death," as a matter of right, or indeed fundamental right? The project here is to examine the phenomenon of self-caused death, especially in the context of physician assistance, with as little ideological baggage as possible.

Is that possible at all? Among opponents of the legalization of the practice of physician-assisted dying, activist Steven Drake has argued against proponents that they are "selling" sanitized language like "aid-in-dying"

---

[2] For a comprehensive sourcebook of historical writings, see Margaret Pabst Battin, ed., *The Ethics of Suicide: Historical Sources* (New York: Oxford University Press, 2015), also available at http://ethicsofsuicide.lib.utah.edu.

as a way of avoiding substantive concerns[3]—an argument that obviously begs the question of whether legalizing assisted "suicide," the term opponents insist on using, is dangerous or wrong. Whether it is possible at all to discuss this issue in fully neutral terms is open to question; even the seemingly unbiased language of "aid in dying" has taken on ideologically tainted positive connotations largely because it is used primarily by proponents of legalizing the practice.

Appeals to rights are ubiquitous on both sides of the social debate. For example, in a case brought in New Mexico in 2014 but typical of legal action everywhere, the state argued that "banning doctor-assisted suicide is consistent with individual rights under the State Constitution"; this same case was decided at the state court level, however, with a ruling by Judge Nan G. Nash that "the liberty, safety and happiness interest of a competent, terminally ill patient to choose aid in dying is a fundamental right under our New Mexico Constitution."[4] Is assisted suicide—aid-in-dying—a *fundamental* right in the view of this judge? She did not offer a philosophically substantive argument for this claim; our project here is to consider whether there may be a plausible one. Note, however, that the judge refers just to a "terminally ill patient"; we must also consider whether a fundamental right to suicide could be broader than this.

The Argument from Dignity and a Linguistic Triple Threat

So here's a way to think of the underlying conceptual issues at stake, and what might ground the claim that "suicide," or rather self-initiated death, is a fundamental right, whether or not terminal illness is the case. This is the argument I made three and a half decades ago; it's in the end about the centrality of *dignity* in the way we might die.

Let us consider the way in which fundamental rights are to be accounted for; here's a quick sketch. Let us take this as a basic premise: *Individuals have fundamental rights to do certain sorts of things just because doing those things tends to be constitutive of human dignity.* "Human dignity," although it is perhaps difficult to define, is nevertheless a notion rooted in

---

[3] Cited in Diane Coleman, "New Mexico Lower Court Parrots the Language and Platitudes of Assisted Suicide Advocacy Groups," *Not Dead Yet News & Commentary*, January 14, 2014, available at http://notdeadyet.org/2014/01/new-mexico-lower-court-parrots-the-language-and-platitudes-of-assisted-suicide-advocacy-groups.html, accessed January 16, 2017.

[4] Erik Eckholm, "New Mexico Judge Affirms Right to 'Aid in Dying'," *New York Times* January 13, 2014: A16. Available at https://www.nytimes.com/2014/01/14/us/new-mexico-judge-affirms-right-to-aid-in-dying.html, accessed January 16, 2017. The case was appealed and denied.

an ideal conception of human life, human community, and human excellence. On this view, although we may take ourselves to have a variety of relatively superficial and easily overridden liberty rights, we also understand ourselves to have more fundamental human rights because we conceive them to establish and promote human dignity. The right freely to associate with others we recognize as a fundamental right because we take free association with others to contribute to our dignity. Alcoholism, on the other hand, for example, does not typically conduce to human dignity; hence, although it may still be a liberty right—namely, when it does not harm other persons—it is not a fundamental right.

Some might indeed argue that a right to suicide is a little like a right to alcoholism: something you have the liberty to do, but not at all necessarily a good thing. But I was arguing for something stronger. While my account of suicide as not just a liberty right but a fundamental one may at first seem to be indeed opportunistic, an ad hoc device for resolving our conflicts about "suicide" or self-initiated death, I believed it would help explain and resolve some of the more volatile disputes concerning other rights and show why there aren't disputes concerning some.

But although this dignity-based account of rights is plausible, I had argued, for fundamental rights in general, it is the particular case of the putative right to suicide, the right to self-initiated death, that makes us notice the central way in which it differs from more conventional accounts. On the account I pursued, *because fundamental rights are rooted in human dignity, they are not equally distributed.* This claim may well seem initially counterintuitive and perhaps morally offensive as well; although we are of course accustomed to assume that liberty rights are unequally distributed (because for different individuals, different special obligations may override them—that is, they are "shaped" to accommodate different inclusions and exclusions), we insist that the distribution of *fundamental* rights is uniform: *All* persons have them, simply in virtue of their being human. But this notion that fundamental rights are equally distributed is an illusion, I argued (although I think it a necessary and desirable one): It reflects not the uniform nature of fundamental rights but, rather, the fact that the things they guarantee tend to be constitutive of human dignity equally for all persons. Liberty is constitutive of dignity for virtually all persons, and for those for whom it is not—small children, for instance, or the incapacitated mentally ill—we recognize the importance of limitations or exceptions. Thus, it may seem to be analytic of the notion of fundamental human rights that they are equally distributed, but it is precisely such cases, especially that of suicide, that show they are not. Some persons in some situations, I attempted to show, have a fundamental right to suicide—that is, to initiate their own deaths; others do not. Of course, the right to suicide, if it is one, is not alone among fundamental rights in being unequally distributed; it is merely more unequally distributed than most. It is this matter of unequal distribution, I claimed, that has disguised from us the fact that being the initiator of one's own death can be a fundamental right.

Does this convoluted account of suicide as a fundamental right succeed? I'm not at all sure about the theoretical argument anymore. Rather, I've come to think that the issue of rights to suicide suffers from a different, largely linguistic set of problems that bedevil clear thinking about the issue in the first place, a kind of philosophic triple threat.

First, there are problems about "rights." As I've said, rights come in a variety of forms: liberty rights, claim rights, legal rights, constitutional rights, derivative rights, and so on; these have been well catalogued by political philosophers and legal theorists over many centuries. The problem here is to identify what precisely the difference is between a liberty right and a fundamental right, beyond the evident fact that we call fundamental rights the sorts of things that turn up in manifestoes. At a minimum, they are things that the authors of a particular manifesto in a particular society regard as more weighty, more important, more worthy of universal recognition, but that doesn't tell us much about how to distinguish comparatively lightweight liberty rights from these heavy-duty ones in the seemingly bizarre claims about suicide.

Second, there are problems about "dignity." My account of fundamental rights was grounded in notions of human dignity, but, as many theorists have pointed out, there are serious difficulties with it. Indeed, writers on dignity have generally left this notion limp and battered, if viable at all: It is used in too many inconsistent ways, co-opted by too many partisans on different sides of ideological debates, and has no incontestably firm roots. If my early account of suicide as a fundamental right does not succeed, perhaps that is in part because the notion of dignity in which it was said to be grounded cannot bear the weight.

But even after reassessing one's earlier position after so many years, I somehow still accept the view that was the original conclusion of this argument, that suicide can (in some cases) be a matter of fundamental right, even if I'm less persuaded of the circuitous argument about unequally distributed rights that I made to establish it. I continue to think that there can be suicides of dignity and that these can be a matter of fundamental right. That's the problem for me to try to explain.

Perhaps my discomfort is associated with Ruth Macklin's famous argument that "dignity is a useless concept."[5] Other authors in this collection have also noted the important role of her claim, and most seem to agree with her that the concept of dignity is, as we might put it, vague, variable, slippery, and so plastic that it is regularly used by both sides in many social arguments—including as we saw in the New Mexico case, the arguments concerning physician-assisted suicide. If you try to ground rights in their contribution to human dignity but you can't really quite pin down what dignity is, your argument teeters on the brink of collapse; just the same, I think, there is still something right about it.

So let's try another tack: a cross-cultural, global view. We can look away from theory for a moment to see what intuitions we might share and what we might have to say about dignity in actual cases. (This is a kind of post-Rawlsian move, to determine if we can square our intuitions with the demands of theory.) Here, too, the picture is not so simple. And it brings us to the third of the linguistic problems that the issue of rights to suicide raises: Exactly what counts as "suicide," anyway?

Any workable account of the role of dignity in suicide—that is, of initiating one's own death—must be able to illuminate a variety of controversial practices, some of which are typically labeled "suicide" but others are labeled "martyrdom" or "self-sacrifice" or various other pejorative or celebratory epithets. These cases too involve initiating or playing a primary causal role in one's own death, but they are not always easy to distinguish from what we label "suicide." Not all cases of suicide involve dignity, no matter how we define it; there are some, perhaps many, clearly catastrophic, needless, awful cases, but that does not yet tell us how to draw a line. Perhaps more telling, there are also cases in which, I think, we fail to perceive elements of dignity—whatever that is—in part because of our background ethical views. For example, we English speakers in the Western world label jihadists "suicide bombers," using the most pejorative term we can; what we fail to see is the element of dignity in a person's choice to use his or her life to defend a faith deeply believed, so masked this element of dignity is both by the possibility of undue influence and, more important, what we understand as the moral wrongness of killing other uninvolved, innocent human beings. We also ignore the fact that "suicide bombers" are never called by that negative term in the culture from which they emerge; there, they are "martyrs." We label the last flights of Japanese kamikaze pilots of World War II "suicide missions," similarly failing—or refusing—to see the

---

[5] Ruth Macklin, "Dignity Is a Useless Concept," *BMJ* 327, no. 7429 (2003):1419–1420.

element of dignity in these young men's choices to honor their emperor, masked from us Western English speakers as the enemy they were attacking. In contrast, we in the West do not as readily label as "suicide" the self-immolations of the Buddhist monks and nuns protesting the Diem regime in Vietnam, or those of monks and nuns protesting Chinese control of Tibet, because our political leanings tend to side with their ideals and the causes for which they undertook to initiate their own deaths; they are martyrs, self-sacrificers, heroes to us, not ordinary suicides. If we do call them suicides, we add that they are "suicides of social protest," thus blunting the negative force of the term "suicide" alone.

Indeed, what counts as "suicide," or something labeled by a term regarded as more ethically acceptable, may appear to be a function of what you see in it. Here, dignity, or something like it, may play a central role, even if not mentioned by name. Consider, for example, Thich Nhat Hanh's explanation of self-immolation to Martin Luther King, Jr., in a letter dated June 1, 1965:

> The self-burning of Vietnamese Buddhist monks in 1963 is somehow difficult for Western Christian conscience to understand. The press spoke then of suicide, but in the essence, it is not. It is not even a protest. What the monks said in the letters they left before burning themselves aimed only at alarming, at moving the hearts of the oppressors, and at calling the attention of the world to the suffering endured then by the Vietnamese. To burn oneself by fire is to prove that what one is saying is of the utmost importance. . . . The Vietnamese monk, by burning himself, says with all his strength and determination that he can endure the greatest of sufferings to protect his people. But why does he have to burn himself to death? The difference between burning oneself and burning oneself to death is only a difference in degree, not in nature. A man who burns himself too much must die. The importance is not to take one's life, but to burn. What he really aims at is the expression of his will and determination, not death. . . . To express will by burning oneself, therefore, is not to commit an act of destruction but perform an act of construction, that is, to suffer and to die for the sake of one's people. This is not suicide. Suicide is an act of self-destruction. . . . The monk believes he is practicing the doctrine of highest compassion by sacrificing himself in order to call the attention of, and to seek help from, the people of the world.[6]

---

[6] Thich Nhat Hanh, *Vietnam: Lotus in a Sea of Fire*, foreword by Thomas Merton (New York: Hill and Wang, 1967), 106–108.

Thich Nhat Hanh does not refer to dignity explicitly; he focuses rather on "compassion," although I sense that many Westerners would ascribe dignity to serious acts of compassion. He also insists that these acts of burning oneself to death are not suicides. One way for Westerners to describe Nhat Hanh's interpretation of these Buddhist monks' acts of self-immolation is to say that he sees only the compassion, the dignity in them—an "act of construction," as he calls it, but not those features that might make others label them suicide. If we were to see what he sees in these self-initiated deaths, the highest expression of dignity—an "act of construction" in choosing to suffer and die for the sake of one's people—we might also naturally speak in terms of rights, thus treading on the ground that dignity can provide for rights. We surely could not imagine claiming these monks and nuns had no right to immolate themselves, or that the quintessentially difficult path they had chosen should have been blocked, or that "suicide prevention" experts should have been called to the scene. In contrast, however, if we saw what the Chinese authorities see in the Tibetan monks and nuns who also immolate themselves—as of this writing, at least 140 have done so—we would see nothing of dignity, but only political agitation and perhaps religious psychopathology, and it would presumably follow that we saw nothing to support any claim about fundamental rights. Indeed, if we saw it from the Chinese authorities' point of view, we would see "violent behaviour whose aim is to create an atmosphere of terror"[7] according to protesters, and we would perhaps even support their policy of suppression.

Part of the point of this discussion is to show that although, as I am maintaining, dignity—whatever that is, or more accurately, whatever range of things it is—is an essential element in that fundamental right to become the author of one's own death. Whether dignity is in fact part of any given individual's "suicidal" action will be open to widely varying interpretations on the part of different observers. Is any particular act of initiating one's own death an "act of destruction," as Thich Nhat Hanh would put it, or an "act of construction"? Whether you are witnessing it from a street corner in Saigon, the railing on the Golden Gate bridge, or in a hospital room in a tertiary medical center somewhere in the high-tech world, and even if you have access to suicide notes, psychological autopsies, and the views of other observers besides yourself, it may still be difficult to tell. The difficulty of answering such a question reinforces Macklin's claim that dignity is a "useless" concept—what counts as dignity to outside

---

[7] See https://www.freetibet.org/field-collection/field-image-section/176, accessed January 7, 2017.

observers is so variable as to be useless in forming public policy or, for that matter, almost any practical application, but the question itself is still open. Is this an act of dignity, or with elements of dignity, or is it an act of desperate, unthinking futility and shame? Dignity, like beauty, may be to a large degree in the eye of the beholder, something to be admired and perhaps emulated, but not objectively real. Just the same, I think it is not only in the beholder's eye.

The deeper problem is that we are working here with not just one but two unstable, slippery terms—"suicide" and "dignity"—a challenge compounded by that third set of difficulties, differentiating types of rights. Our nomenclature distorts our perceptions, but our perceptions are colored by extraneous circumstances and matters of background cultural socialization. For example, how do we differentiate suicide from martyrdom? This is a traditional challenge for Judaism, Christianity, and Islam—and they all do it in slightly different ways. What counts as dignity in various world cultures, or even subcultures close to home? How are liberty rights and fundamental rights distinguished in the various cultures throughout the world, if rights are even recognized at all? Here, too, varying cultures recognize conceptions of something that could be called dignity, but they do it in different ways.

We also label acts "suicide," or on the contrary some honorific term such as "heroism," on different underlying grounds: Sometimes it's the causal route from self-initiation to death; sometimes it's the intention under which the causal route to death is put in gear. For example, we would call the depressed person who drives his car over a cliff a "suicide" but the pilot of a failing jet who crashes it in an empty field to avoid a crowded schoolyard a "hero," even though each controlled the causal route that led to his death. What's at the root of this problem, I think, is that the concepts of "dignity" and "suicide" co-vary; they each have multiple meanings, but those meanings vary inversely in relation to each other. We readily say of self-sacrificial and heroic acts that are fatal that they are infused with dignity; on the other hand, if we call it "suicide," we dismiss it as warped, emotionally overwrought, pathological, tragic behavior. "Suicide" is, in short, a concept negatively related to "dignity" in contexts in which they both appear. To put it in a more elementary way, in the popular understanding "dignity" just doesn't go with "suicide," and "suicide" has nothing to do with "dignity." If it is a self-initiated death we admire, we call it by those other honorific terms; if it is a self-initiated death we don't admire, then it's suicide. Thus, we can't really talk about these issues in stable terms. That's at least part of why we can't seem to answer the question posed here: *What's the role of human dignity in assisted suicide?* It's a triple threat to cogent discussion; we might as well say that this challenge is posing an impossible, unanswerable question.

But I think that's wrong and that the question asked here is not in its content an unanswerable one. I still have the sense that a right, a fundamental right, to suicide is grounded somehow in human dignity.

Let me remark parenthetically that this problem may be more entrenched for speakers of some languages than others. English, as I've pointed out elsewhere,[8] has just one principal term for the act in question, *suicide*; it is supported by various more specific causal expressions, such as hanging oneself or drowning oneself or shooting oneself in the head, but these are all understood as varieties of suicide. German, in contrast, has four terms in ubiquitous use: *Selbstmord* (lit. self-murder), *Selbstötung* (lit. self-killing), *Suizid* (the Latinate form)—the popular, bureaucratic, and medical terms, all with varying degrees of negative connotation—and one that is more positively and romantically valenced, *Freitod* (lit. free death). This is just to say that German speakers are able to have this conversation about "suicide" and dignity in a more linguistically nimble way than English speakers can; we English speakers are always stuck with the heavy moral baggage that our one main term for self-initiated death normally carries.

Let's try yet another tack, in which the label "suicide" is used but there are nevertheless issues of dignity. Consider the case of Sofia, a seventy-nine-year-old Swedish woman who in 2013 took a lethal dose of pills while her family was on its summer vacation. It's a case in which the causal route is clear, but because we have only one informant and that information is transmitted through someone committed to a favorable view of "death with dignity," we cannot really know the intention under which the agent acted. Sofia died without telling her family, including her fifteen-year-old grandson, or her physician, or with one exception anyone else about her plan:

> The family was appalled about her suicide. To them, she was a dear mother and a beloved grandmother, and she was not severely ill. The son found her, after returning from a summer vacation. The grandson, particularly, who was 15, went into a mental state—he loved his grandmother very much. Everybody, the family, the neighbors, the relatives, were outraged. They

---

[8] Margaret Pabst Battin, "Assisted Suicide: What Can We Learn from Germany?", in *The Least Worst Death* (New York: Oxford University Press, 1994), 254–270.

contacted Sofia's house doctor, who knew nothing. They accused the RTVD [the Swedish right-to-die society] of leading her astray.

At RTVD, however, Sofia had found a friend who had her confidence. She knew of Sofia's reasoning. The two had long talks about dying. Sofia's planning started many years earlier. She bought books from abroad and googled the Internet. She bought the right kind of pills from a foreign country. They were in a safe, cool and dark place. They were of great comfort to her.

Sofia was not sick, although she had a number of ailments, common at her age. She lived alone, most of her friends were dead and she seldom saw her relatives. Most of the time, she was alone. There was no suffering. Neither did she see any point in continuing life when her future was running out.

In Sweden, there is no understanding whatsoever about suicides, not even for old people with a mortal disease. Even the normal death is hidden away as much as possible. She concluded it was not possible to discuss her thoughts in the family. They would feel the need to stop her, or else to be responsible. To Sofia, they would be a burden when all she wanted was to concentrate only on her own feelings. This was her death. She expected no one to have to share it with her. The choice was hers and hers alone.

In this respect, her reasoning was considerate. She meant to be fully responsible for her own death. Sofia knew she must not postpone things too long. Her mind was still clear, and she knew what she was doing. She could by no means know whether she would get a stroke or something similar to prevent her plans. She needed to be alone for 10–12 hours, so as not to be found too early. That is why she chose the time when the family was on summer leave. The evening she took her pills, she felt prepared, calm and without regrets. She was at peace.

But Sofia's considerations were not appreciated. Her family, her few friends, her neighbors—they were shocked, they were outraged and furious. How could she be so selfish? How could she think only of herself? What about them? What about their feelings?[9]

A most important characteristic of dignity, I had argued in my earlier paper, is a characteristic of the individual in relation to his or her world: It is that one cannot promote one's own dignity by destroying the dignity

---

[9] Berit Hasselmark, "The Selfish Suicide?", *World Right-to-Die Newsletter*, no. 65 (December 2013): 8, available at http://www.worldrtd.net/sites/default/files/newsfiles/WRTD%20 Newsletter%201213Web.pdf, accessed January 16, 2017.

of someone else, although one can certainly promote one's own interests, happiness, or reputation at another's expense. If I try to elevate my dignity by robbing you of yours, I lose my own as well—even though I may nevertheless gain happiness, satisfaction of my interests, and other self-enhancing benefits. Thus, I had argued then, the concept of dignity is not wholly empirical but contains ideal features as well. Now, however, I see that it is a good deal more slippery than I'd thought.

So what of Sofia's suicide while her family was on its summer vacation, a time she reportedly picked to minimize the possibility of being discovered? It is reported that the family members were angry and devastated, especially the fifteen-year-old grandson. Do these harms which Sofia's suicide caused them preclude thinking of her self-initiated death as an act of dignity? What, precisely, were her intentions in taking this route, and do they in any case matter to a moral assessment of her act?

Two entirely different views are possible here: one, that her act was selfish and cruel to those around her; and the other, that her act was reflective, rational, and deeply considerate of others in that it would not put them in guilt-fostering situations of trying to intervene and would preclude her ever becoming a burden to them. Do we know which one is correct? Virtually no amount of comment from outsiders will determine this; what they see in this case will be largely a function of their antecedent views. Indeed, my guess is that it was both; but we do not have the linguistic flexibility to say that her suicide was both an act of dignity and an act of indignity; the very concept of dignity seems to function in a way that is largely indivisible, and it makes little sense of such an assessment.

What, then, about the issue of dignity and physician-assisted suicide, or euthanasia, or, more neutrally phrased, physician-aided dying or medical aid in dying? Jihadists, kamikaze pilots, Buddhist monks and nuns, and the seventy-nine-year-old Swedish woman Sofia were all the agents of their own deaths, and they acted without the assistance of a physician. But what about dignity and fundamental rights at the bedside of the terminally ill or the chronically ill or disabled, people who choose to die but for whom the policy issue is whether they have such a right? There are issues of causation and intention involved, playing out against the triply unstable background in our understandings of rights, dignity, and suicide.

Let me portray for you the situation of one individual with whom I've been closely acquainted (to say the least) and for whom I was among and directed those providing care. I provide this case because I was closer than anyone else to observing causal routes, intentions, and other factors that might shape our thinking. A double-bicycle collision had in one split second rendered this previously healthy, athletic man quadriplegic, ventilator-dependent, and in need of complete care for all bodily functions; injured at C2/C3, he had virtually no movement below the tops of his shoulders. This meant all cleaning and bathing had to be done by others; all feeding had to be done manually by others; if a spot on his face itched, it had to be scratched by others. It meant lifting his 6-foot, 5-inch body by means of a hoist to a motorized wheelchair and back again. It meant frequent and regular pulmonary suction, bringing secretions up through his tracheostomy that he was unable to cough out himself. It meant urinary catheterization every four hours, around the clock, and it meant he could never be alone, requiring a trained caregiver in the room with him, within earshot, or within range of a baby monitor that transmitted every sound, lest there be a pulmonary crisis that could block his breathing in a matter of minutes. There was frequent, sometimes severe, pain. He required diapers, delicately called "briefs." And, in the procedure that was most likely to be described as an affront to dignity, he required manual digital stimulation of the rectum, every day, as one of his twelve different caregivers inserted their gloved fingers to induce his bowels to move. Yet he had had no brain injury in the bicycle accident, and he was fully and completely lucid and aware all the time he was receiving this care.

Some former friends could hardly bear to see him this way, reduced as they saw him from the vigorous, active man he had been. Others who did visit were moved by the pain, limitation, and constant effort to endure the various medical and nursing procedures his condition involved. And, much to the point of this discussion of rights at the end of life, almost all of them—including me—said at one point or another that they "didn't think they could do what he was doing"—that is, live in this situation; they would rather that the accident, if it had to occur at all, had been fatal on the spot.

Were they responding only to the very considerable physical suffering his condition involved? Or were they responding to something more central, the loss of freedom, autonomy, liberty of choice and movement his situation seemed to entail? At the same time, however, many cherished their human interaction with him: He was lucid, reflective, intellectually stimulating, and as far as his brain went, functioning at a new and even more challenging level, beyond what an ordinary English professor might achieve. In many ways, he flourished—his friendships grew deeper, his relationships with family enhanced, his love for his wife (me) intensified and was returned in intensified kind. Friends came from everywhere; he taught courses; and he and I kept a running account of our joint experience in this unfathomably new situation.[10] We insisted that it was only a tragedy if we let it be that way. No one, however moved they were by his sufferings, ever as far as I know questioned his dignity, at least not to me; indeed, in many ways seeing his sufferings seemed for some observers to enhance it.

But, after repeated pneumonias and infections with many of the microbes a hospital has to offer, things began to deteriorate. He talked about dying. He talked about his fears of dying, of how he might die, but as time went on he said more and more insistently that he wanted to die. Was this a loss of dignity, a decline into what Thich Nhat Hanh later in the same letter defines as suicide, "an act of self-destruction, having as causes the following: (1) lack of courage to live and to cope with difficulties; (2) defeat by life and loss of all hope; (3) desire for nonexistence"? How could we possibly tell, even with the most probing psychotherapeutic assessment? In the end, he did choose to die, making a formal request to have his ventilator removed, and securing the assistance of a hospice physician to do so. He was clearly within his legal rights to have medical therapies he no longer wanted discontinued. But was this within his *fundamental* rights, rooted in the dignity of this individual human being, a choice to be accorded the fullest, if most painful, respect? It was regarded as "noble," "heroic," and indeed an act of consummate dignity by most of his friends, his acquaintances, and by many commentators in the public media coverage of this story. I even heard the term "bodhisattva" used of him by a Buddhist monk who knew him well.

But not everyone saw it this way. Indeed, were it not for the publicly conspicuous happenstance of having a ventilator and four other life-prolonging devices, if he were just another ordinary patient who seemed to give up, for whom the burdens of illness and limitation had come to outweigh the benefits of remaining alive, would it have been regarded as simple suicide? Were it not for the life-prolonging technology and thus the legal opportunity to discontinue them, the assistance of a physician would not have been legal in the jurisdiction in which he lived, and the act itself might have been viewed in a much less heroic way, indeed, unfortunate perhaps and pitiable, but not at all dignified in any real sense. Indeed, it seems, in end-of-life contexts, the background medical situation, the legal

---

[10] Brooke Hopkins and Peggy Battin, *Love under Trial*, manuscript based on account at www.brookeandpeggy.blogspot.com. Also see Robin Marantz Henig, "A Life or Death Situation," *The New York Times Magazine*, July 21, 2013, available at http://www.nytimes.com/2013/07/21/magazine/a-life-or-death-situation.html?hp&_r=0.

status of an action, and even its "ordinariness" can play a role in whether a life-ending act is perceived as an act of dignity or not; these adventitious circumstances may play a role in whether it is recognized as suicide or self-sacrifice, suicide or heroism, or suicide or one of the most difficult but noble acts of which humankind is capable at all.

Dignity, Suicide, and Terminal Illness

Let me skip over the case of "ordinary" terminal illness, the context of physician-assisted suicide, or, as supporters prefer to say, physician aid-in-dying. It seems to me simply obvious to say that some "suicides" in these circumstances are indeed suicides of dignity, "acts of construction" in facing the unavoidable end of one's life, whereas others are desperate, fearful, entirely self-focused acts of destruction, seeking only to obliterate that locus of pain and suffering, one's own self. Most, I venture, have some elements of both. Dare we say they are both undignified and dignified at the same time? Negative and positive dignity appraisals seem to be mutually exclusive in ordinary use and do not admit of partial application; to say that an act is both undignified and dignified seems to make no sense, although I believe that is often the case.

Dignity, Suicide, and Old Age

Rather, looking ahead, let us turn instead to a more difficult problem, one now coming into focus in discussions in the United Kingdom and the Netherlands in particular. It is the issue of suicide in old age, or as in the (former) name of one of the societies supporting such practices, "old age rational suicide," or SOARS.[11] It is often described as the choice to die by older people who are "tired of life" or "through with life," people whom a student of mine once dubbed "sufficiently satisfied seniors."[12] Can there

---

[11] The Society for Old Age Rational Suicide, founded in the United Kingdom in 2009, changed its name in 2016 to "My Death, My Decision" (MDMD). The organization's website explains, "This reflects a broadening of objectives beyond 'old age,' and an acceptance that for most people in the UK, the word 'suicide' is inextricably linked with tragic, emotional, lonely and often violent loss of life. This is in stark contrast to the type of voluntary, medically assisted death we campaign for—a peaceful, well considered, individual choice, following professional counselling, possibly in the company of friends and relatives. MDMD believe this should be a legally available option to mentally competent adults, whose quality of life is permanently reduced below the level they are able to accept, due to medical conditions where there is little or no chance of meaningful recovery." See http://www.soars.org.uk, accessed January 17, 2017.

[12] This point was made in oral conversation by Stevenson Smith.

be dignity in these self-willed, self-initiated deaths? First, is there any general principle, either beyond those already invoked in the current debate about physician-assisted dying, or any subsidiary or alternative principle specific to the situation of suicide in old age, absent terminal illness, that might speak to this issue? I know of none. Bracket all the usual concerns, among them whether it would harm immediate others such as family and friends, or whether it would weaken the social fabric, whether it would undermine the physician–patient relationship or compromise the integrity of the physician; whether it would constitute an affront to the State or to God. Bracket also the question of whether it would open the floodgates to abuse. These are the standard concerns about physician-assisted dying in any context, but they do not address the distinctive situation of old age. Can we imagine the older person surveying her past, her present, and the future that awaits her as an aging person? Can we imagine it as an act of dignity for her to choose to end her life now, not in secrecy as the Swedish woman Sofia felt she had to do, but with the assent of her family and friends, the loyal assistance of her physician, an act supported by social and legal structures as one among the full range of choices an older person may lawfully make about how to live out the end of a finite life?

Consider the account given by Valerius Maximus, the Roman writer who was attached to the retinue of Sextus Pompeius (consul and later proconsul of Asia during the reign of the emperor Tiberius and part of a literary circle to which Ovid belonged), and who accompanied Sextus to the East in the mid-20s AD. In *Memorable Doings and Sayings*, Valerius writes first of the Massilians, inhabitants of what is now Marseilles, and then of a ninety-year-old woman on the island of Cea:

> A poison compounded of hemlock is under public guard in that community which is given to one who has shown reasons to the Six Hundred, as their senate is called, why death is desirable for him. The enquiry is conducted with firmness tempered by benevolence, not suffering the subject to leave life rashly but providing swift means of death to one who rationally desires a way out. Thus persons encountering an excess of bad fortune or good (for either might afford reason for ending life, the one lest it continue, the other lest it fail) find a finish to it in an approved departure.
>
> I believe this usage of the Massilians did not originate in Gaul but was borrowed from Greece because I saw it also observed in the island of Cea when I entered the town of Iulis on my way to Asia with Sex. Pompeius. For it so happened on that occasion that a lady of the highest rank there but in extreme old age, after explaining to her fellow citizens why she ought to

depart from life, determined to put an end to herself by poison and set much store on having her death gain celebrity by the presence of Pompeius. Nor could that gentleman reject her plea, excellently endowed as he was with the virtue of good nature as with all other noble qualities. So he visited her and in fluent speech, which flowed from his lips as from some copious fountain of eloquence, tried at length but in vain to turn her back from her design. Finally he let her carry out her intention. Having passed her ninetieth year in the soundest health of mind and body, she lay on her bed, which was spread, as far as might be perceived, more elegantly than every day, and resting on her elbow she spoke: "Sex. Pompeius, may the gods whom I am leaving rather than those to whom I am going repay you because you have not disdained to urge me to live nor yet to be witness of my death. As for me, I have always seen Fortune's smiling face. Rather than be forced through greed of living to see her frown, I am exchanging what remains of my breath for a happy end, leaving two daughters and a flock of seven grandchildren to survive me." Then, having urged her family to live in harmony, she distributed her estate among them, and having consigned her own observance and the domestic rites to her elder daughter, she took the cup in which the poison had been mixed in a firm grasp. After pouring libations to Mercury and invoking his divine power, that he conduct her on a calm journey to the happier part of the underworld, she eagerly drained the fatal potion. She indicated in words the parts of her body which numbness seized one by one, and when she told us that it was about to reach her vitals and heart, she summoned her daughters' hands to the last office, to close her eyes. As for us Romans, she dismissed us, stunned by so extraordinary a spectacle but bathed in tears.[13]

What is notable about Valerius' account is his report that two sorts of reasons were recognized as compelling for ending one's life: if one faced severe suffering or other hardships, or if one's life were going really well and one did not choose to face a later decline. It is the latter in particular that raises the issue of dignity in suicide in old age: whether preemptive suicide, undertaken at that time when one might be described as a "sufficiently satisfied senior," might be a moment of particular dignity when one clearly foresees, but elects not to undergo, the downward slide that is characteristic of aging. Given the graying of so many nations, our own included, and the rapid rise in the proportions of older people to young

---

[13] Valerius Maximus, *Memorable Doings and Sayings*, Book II, ed. and trans. D. R. Shackleton Bailey (Cambridge, Mass.: Harvard University Press, 2000), 167–177.

ones, this is I think *the* mortality issue for our immediate future, even if the language in which we discuss it is vague, variable, slippery, and so plastic that it can be used by both sides in many social arguments, including this very one. That we cannot say exactly what should count as "suicide," that we cannot pin down a precise account of "dignity," and that we don't even know what rights to invoke should not dissuade us from facing a consummately important issue like this—recognizing, however inchoately, that the question of dignity must be a central element of it. Can we imagine a choice like that of the ninety-year-old woman of Cea visited by Sextus Pompeius becoming recognized as the noble, heroic, ideal model for societies of the future, "leave while you're ahead, not after Fortune begins to play you false"?—this I think is the mortality issue of the future we will have to face—and should face, both conceptually and in practice. It would radically change the way we think about the end of life, and of course sweep the issues of self-initiated and physician-assisted dying into a new vortex of ethical controversy along with it.

The Upshot

What's the upshot of this discussion? I'd begun so optimistically those three and a half decades ago thinking it would be possible to provide a somewhat rigorous theoretical account of the role of dignity and rights in issues about suicide; part of the point of doing so was to provide the conceptual structure that would permit a Rawlsian-flavored back-and-forth, pruning-and-adjusting attempt to reach some form of reflective equilibrium concerning the claim that suicide is a matter of fundamental right. That part of the project, providing a rigorous theoretical account of dignity, rights, and suicide, now seems unrealistically optimistic, indeed, one might say, naive, vulnerable to the triple linguistic threat. In this set of further explorations I've pursued a rather different tack, examining a variety of different cases, including historical, cross-cultural, current, and direct-experience examples that would have been the other pole of a reflective-equilibrium project. This part isn't working either; what I see is too many different "intuitions" about these cases, often starkly different, hardly a basis for the civilized sort of pruning-and-adjusting between theory and intuitions about cases that Rawls had in mind.

But just because it isn't working doesn't mean there isn't something there. I still think there is. And I also think that because this attempt isn't yielding the kind of firm answer one might have sought, it just means that the issue is more complex, more fractured, but therefore also more interesting than we might have realized in advance. We will surely see more tension in our theories and disagreements in practice about this issue as we and our societies continue to age, and as we each begin to face the deaths we have ahead.

CHAPTER 13 | Human Dignity and the Right
to Assisted Suicide

HOLGER BAUMANN AND PETER SCHABER

Introduction

What is the role of human dignity in discussions about assisted suicide? In the following, we argue that it yields an argument in favor of the moral permissibility of assisted suicide. If a person competently requests another person to assist her in dying, she thereby exercises her normative power to make the act permissible. Denying a person this normative power means to disrespect her human dignity. We thus argue against views that regard terminating one's own life (by the help of others) as morally impermissible for reasons of human dignity. At the same time, however, we depart from views according to which human dignity delivers reasons or puts other persons under a duty to help a person terminate her life. On our view, then, appeals to human dignity yield neither a duty nor even reasons to help. Respect for human dignity with regard to the practice of assisted suicide only amounts to the claim that we should respect a person's normative power to make assisting acts morally permissible.

In arguing for these claims, in the first part of this chapter, we develop a version of a status-based conception of human dignity. Such conceptions contrast with value-based conceptions in that they have a deontic rather than axiological basis. An influential account of the latter can be found in Kant, who holds that beings with dignity have "absolute worth." In contrast to things or beings that have only relative worth, Kant argues that beings with absolute worth do not have a price, by which he means not only that they have no market price but also that they do not allow to be replaced by an equivalent or to be compared with the value of another thing: "What has a price can be replaced by something as its equivalent; what on the other hand is raised above all price and therefore admits of no equivalent has dignity."[1] Following Kant, the notion of dignity is often characterized in the debate as follows: Beings with human dignity have absolute worth, and to respect their dignity means to honor their worth; if we put a price on beings with dignity and, for example, compare the value of lives of persons, we thus show disrespect for their dignity. In the context of self-determination, David Velleman has prominently argued in a Kantian fashion that it is never morally permissible to terminate one's own life because it can never be the case that the amount of a person's suffering outweighs the absolute value that persons themselves have.[2]

In order to make plausible why we pursue a status-based conception in this chapter, we raise one general worry with regard to such value-based conceptions of dignity at this point. The general question we regard as important is the following: Does a value-based conception provide us with an understanding of human dignity that helps to explain why we regard certain acts such as degradation and humiliation as paradigmatic violations of human dignity? It might be claimed that such actions are instances of not honoring the absolute worth of a person. However, the wrongness of humiliating a person does not seem to consist in assigning a price to her—it does not amount to comparing her value or to replacing her with an equivalent. It is thus unclear how the notion of an absolute worth helps us to make sense of the distinctive wrongness of instances of degradation or humiliation.

In our view, the alternative approach to human dignity as a moral status fares initially better with regard to such paradigmatic violations of human dignity. On status-based accounts, dignity is understood as a status that is closely connected to having and exercising rights. Violations of human dignity are violations of legitimate claims of persons rather than instances of not honoring their (absolute) value. Jeremy Waldron has put forward such a view.[3] Although the notion of status was historically related to hierarchy and different social roles and claims, Waldron argues that human dignity should be understood as a universalized high rank and a legal status of being a right-bearer. We draw upon his approach but argue that dignity is first and foremost a *moral* (not a legal) status and that the notion of

---

[1] Immanuel Kant, *Grounding for the Metaphysics of Morals. On a Supposed Right to Lie Because of Philanthropic Concerns*, trans. James W. Ellington, 3rd ed. (Indianapolis, Ind.: Hackett, 1993).
[2] See J. David Velleman, "A Right of Self-Termination?", *Ethics* 109, no. 3 (1999): 606–628.
[3] See Jeremy Waldron, *Dignity, Rank, and Rights* (New York: Oxford University Press, 2012).

normative powers plays a central role in characterizing this status: Very roughly, to have and to exercise normative powers means to be someone who can and is allowed to competently exercise, and in particular waive, her rights. Violations of human dignity are instances in which persons are treated as if they have no say in what may be done to them—that is, in which they are denied their normative powers. As we hope to show in detail in the following sections, such a conception can make better moral sense of humiliation and degradation.[4]

Drawing on this general account, in the second part of this chapter, we apply it to the case of assisted suicide and argue that a person in this case exercises her normative power to waive her right to life that is linked to a bundle of rights over her own body. We also explain why, as stated previously, appeals to human dignity only create permissions for other persons in the case of assisted suicide. This enables us to locate our argument within the debate of assisted suicide and to clarify the distinct role and normative function of dignity. In particular, it helps to understand the relation of human dignity and the argument from autonomy and to understand the importance of other arguments that appeal, for example, to unbearable suffering. Such arguments, we contend, might provide us with *reasons* (or even a duty) to help other persons—reasons that cannot be delivered by human dignity alone.

Normative Powers

In order to introduce the idea of dignity as a moral status, it is instructive to examine the idea of a legal status. A person has such a status if she has certain rights that are guaranteed by the legal system.[5] Together with those rights, persons are also granted certain normative powers that belong to the rights in question. Now, in some cases, normative powers are related to specific social roles or responsibilities. Take, for example, the normative powers that come with being a judge. A judge has the right and power to administer the law and can, for example, send someone to prison. The sentence is an exercise of the normative powers the judge has, and it is authoritative for members of the respective legal community. His verdict puts executives under a duty to restrict the freedom of the convict, and it puts

---

[4] Parts of this chapter draw on ideas developed in Peter Schaber, "Würde als Status," in *Menschenwürde. Eine philosophische Debatte über Dimensionen ihrer Kontingenz*, ed. Eva Guskar-Weber and Mario Brandhorst (Berlin: Suhrkamp, 2017, 45–59).

[5] See Waldron, *Dignity, Rank, and Rights*, 134.

other members of the community under a duty to accept this restriction. Although the imprisonment was illegitimate before the judge's verdict, it is now obligatory. This is, to put it in a general way, how normative powers work and what they do: They change the deontic status of acts.

If we talk about the dignity of the judge that is to be respected, we mean that the normative powers that derive from the role of being a judge have to be respected—that is, that he or she can administer law and thereby put other members of the legal community under a duty. Of course, the judge's dignity is not the same as human dignity. It is a form of contingent dignity because it is socially ascribed and can be lost again. In contrast, human beings have dignity not because of a certain social role but, rather, because they are human beings with certain properties and a certain normative standing. This dignity cannot be lost. What is illuminating for thinking about human dignity, however, is that it can also be regarded as a status that is connected with normative powers. To be someone with dignity means, or so we argue, to have normative powers to change the deontic status of actions—to make, for example, actions permissible that are impermissible without the exercise of our normative powers.

Such normative powers belong to certain rights that we have over ourselves. Without having rights, then, we would have no normative powers. We need not settle the question at this point why persons have such rights or what rights persons have. We assume that as persons we have, for example, rights over our own bodies and our own thoughts, and also over what may be done with our bodies and thoughts. Such rights are understood as moral rights (that might translate into legal rights but do not have to), and they imply corresponding duties on the part of other persons. To illustrate our idea, consider the right not to be touched by other persons: Persons have such a right, and others thus have a corresponding duty not to touch them. Anyone who does not comply with this duty violates a right persons have and thus wrongs them. Now, the right not to be touched is linked to the normative power to waive this right. If a person allows someone to touch her, she thereby releases the other person from a duty and grants her a privilege—something she may do without being obliged to do it.[6] However, it is important to note that by exercising the normative power,

---

[6] The idea of having normative powers to waive rights and grant privileges was originally developed by Wesley N. Hohfeld; see Wesley N. Hohfeld, *Fundamental Legal Conceptions as Applied in Judicial Reasoning*, ed. by D. Campbell and P. Thomas, with an introduction by N. E. Simmonds (Aldershot, UK: Ashgate, 2001). See also Neil MacCormick and Joseph Raz, "Voluntary Obligations and Normative Powers," *Proceedings of the Aristotelian Society. Supplementary Volumes* 46, no. 1 (1972): 59–102.

she does not give up her right. In particular, the other person does not obtain a right to touch her intimately; she only gets a permission to do something.

By consenting to an act, then, a person exercises her normative power. This is only possible if she has normative power over the act in question. It is controversial whether all rights that we have over our own person are related to normative powers to waive these rights. For example, it might be claimed that we have no power to give other persons a permission to torture or to enslave us. However, it is commonly assumed that *most* rights are related to normative powers in the way that we have described in this section, and as we argue next, we would not be persons with dignity if we had no such normative powers.

Moral Wrongness and Violations of Human Dignity

We have suggested that if a person's rights are violated by someone without her permission, she is morally wronged. Are all rights violations also violations of human dignity? In our view, this is not the case. Whether a person shows disrespect for the dignity of another person depends on the normative beliefs that guide her rights-violating acts. What constitutes a dignity violation is the fact that the action is guided by the belief that the victim has no say in determining what may be done to her and that her consent is thus not required. In other words, the dignity of a person is violated if she is treated as if she had no normative power over her rights.

Consider the following example: If Laura touches Paul without his consent, Laura violates Paul's right over his own body. But Laura does not have to entertain the belief that Paul has no right not to be touched—she could touch him without his consent and still have the belief that Paul may not be touched without his consent. In this case, Laura would violate Paul's right, but she would not violate his dignity. If, however, Laura touched Paul without his consent, thinking that she can do as she pleases and that no consent is required, she would violate Paul's dignity. She would then treat him as if he had no say in determining what may be done to him.

In our view, violations of human dignity should be understood along these lines: A person is being treated in ways that deny her the standing of being a person with rights and normative powers. The most radical and severe form of violating a person's dignity, on this account, is to treat her in ways that are guided by the belief that she has no say at all in how she may be treated by others. In such cases, the person would be treated like a slave—that is, as a person who has no normative powers at all. However, as stated previously, dignity violations also occur in less global scenarios, namely in all instances in which a person is denied her normative powers. In the following section, we explain in more detail why this account of human dignity allows us to understand why exactly degradation and humiliation are commonly regarded as paradigmatic violations of human dignity. We take this to be an important reason to understand dignity as having the moral status of having normative powers—that is, of being able to waive one's rights.

Normative Powers and Paradigmatic Violations of Human Dignity

Let us start with an example of a humiliating action: Consider a prison officer who commands a prisoner to come close so that he can wipe his dirty shoes on the prisoner's trousers. The prisoner cannot defend himself and has to helplessly endure the procedure. The harm that is done to the prisoner is marginal here. And clearly, the prison officer does not primarily attempt to harm him. His action is rather symbolical: He wants to demonstrate that the prisoner has no say in what may be done to him. By dominating him, the prison officer conveys the message that the prisoner has no normative standing: "I may do to you whatever I want." It is not the right violation that constitutes the humiliation. It is the denial of the normative powers of the prisoner that turns it into a violation of human dignity.

Acts of humiliation, we assume, are paradigmatic violations of human dignity: They not only violate the rights of persons but also do so in a way that unequivocally gives expression to the belief that the other person has no normative powers to determine what may to be done to her. It is important to emphasize this point because the close connection between violations of rights and violations of human dignity has led some philosophers to the view that having human dignity amounts to having rights and to make claims on others to fulfill the corresponding duties. Joel Feinberg, for example, writes,

> Having rights enables us to "stand up like men," to look others in the eye, and to feel in some fundamental way the equal of anyone. . . . Indeed, respect for persons . . . may simply be respect for their rights, so that there cannot be the one without the other; and what is called "human dignity" may simply be the recognizable capacity to assert claims. To respect a person then, or to

think of him as possessed of human dignity, simply *is* to think of him as a potential maker of claims.[7]

According to Feinberg, we should conceive of human dignity as the capacity to make claims on others—that is, to be able to demand that other persons do not violate one's rights and comply with their duties. However, it seems misleading to link human dignity to the capacity to make claims. Right-holders may be unable to claim their rights in certain situations—for example, because they are intimidated. We should thus better understand Feinberg as saying that human dignity denotes the *entitlement* to make claims on others—an entitlement that is in place even if the person is currently not capable of demanding from others to comply with their duties. But even if we interpret Feinberg in this way, it seems that his account does not capture the distinctiveness of violations of human dignity. Although having rights and being entitled to make claims on others is a necessary condition for having dignity, his theory fails to take into account the central element of human dignity—that is, the possession of normative powers.

To make this idea more clear, imagine a world in which persons have rights but no normative powers.[8] Other persons would have the duty not to violate their rights—for example, not to touch them intimately. Without normative powers, however, persons would be unable to waive their rights and to give other persons permissions. They could thus not release others from their duties and determine what may be done to them. As a consequence, we contend, we would no longer be able to make sense of the distinctive character and wrongness of humiliating actions. Certainly, the prison officer in the example given previously violates a right of the prisoner. He thereby violates his duty to respect the prisoner's rights. But this is not the reason why we think he violates the dignity of the prisoner. He does so by treating him as if the prisoner had no say in how he may be treated. He humiliates him by denying his normative powers.

---

[7] See Joel Feinberg, "The Nature and Value of Rights," *Journal of Value Inquiry* 4, no. 4 (1970): 243–257, 252.

[8] This is, of course, a variation of Feinberg's famous thought experiment of "Nowheresville," a "virtuous world without rights." In a similar vein, Meyers argues that in a world in which persons have rights but lack control over themselves, they would not have human dignity. Our suggestion to understand this objection is to say that if persons have no normative powers that belong to rights, they lack human dignity. See Michael Meyers, "Dignity, Rights, and Self-Control," *Ethics* 99, no. 3 (1989): 520–534.

In summary, we hold that actions are humiliating because they are expressive of the view that the person concerned has no say in what may be done to her. In order to be able to determine what others may do to us, we need more than rights; we need normative powers. They are not recognized by the prison guard. He rather behaves as if he can set the law of what may or may not be done with the prisoner.

Normative Powers and Autonomy

At this point, one might object that the account of human dignity given previously renders the concept redundant because human dignity means nothing else than respect for autonomy or the right to live an autonomous life.[9] After all, it seems that we hold that a person's dignity is violated if her will is disregarded as normatively irrelevant and that a person's dignity is respected if her will is assigned normative importance. The examples considered above might be read as supporting this claim—both touching someone intimately without his or her consent and using someone in the way the prison officer does could be understood as instances of disrespect for the autonomy of the victims.

However, this conclusion is premature. To begin with, the account we have outlined is based on the notion of moral rights that are related to normative powers to exercise these rights. Without having a right, a person's will is not normatively relevant. Think of Paul again, who could autonomously want that Laura gets intimate with him. Imagine that he fulfills all conditions that are set out by different accounts of autonomy; for example, he identifies with his first-order desire to be touched on a higher order, he has developed this desire in an autonomy-preserving way, and the desire rationally coheres with other desires or commitments of him—it is, then, a desire that is "fully his own" in any imaginable sense. What allows Laura to touch Paul, however, is not that he (autonomously) wants to be touched by her. What allows her to touch Paul is his consent. By consenting, he is waiving his right not to be touched by others. In other words, it is the exercise of the normative power that releases Laura from her duty.

That our account of human dignity differs from an autonomy account of dignity is also supported by the following thought: Paul could allow Laura to touch him without wanting to be touched by her. One can allow others to do things that one does not want them to do. You could even

---

[9] See Ruth Macklin, "Dignity Is a Useless Concept," *BMJ* 327, no. 7429 (2003): 1419–1420.

hope that they would not do it.[10] Paul thus only needs to *want to make the action permissible*—he does not have to want that the action be performed. Consent has a normative force as an exercise of normative power, not as an act of wanting others to do something. Of course, the will to make it permissible has to be his will and thus fulfill the conditions that have to be met to call Paul's will his own will. The normative work, however, is done by the exercise of the normative power, not by his autonomous will.

Human Dignity and the Moral Permissibility of Assisted Suicide

We have argued that human dignity should be understood with reference to the moral status of persons to have normative powers that enable them to exercise their rights and change the deontic status of actions. We have also discussed why this account is, in our view, especially well-suited to explain why humiliating and degrading actions are commonly regarded as paradigmatic violations of human dignity—their point is exactly to deny a person's normative standing of having a say in how he or she may be treated. Finally, we have argued that our account is different from autonomy accounts of dignity. Having normative powers to waive a right and make an action permissible is not the same as autonomously deciding to take that action.

Against this background, we are now in a position to develop our claim that human dignity makes assisted suicide morally permissible, but neither creates a duty nor even reasons for other persons to assist a person in terminating her life. In other words, we hold that the role of human dignity with regard to the practice of assisted suicide is in an important regard more limited than is believed by those who claim that "not to assist me in dying is a violation of my human dignity!" On our view, appeals to human dignity should rather take the following form: "To deny me the authority to make permissible that other persons assist me in terminating my own life, and thus to treat me as someone who has no say in determining what may be done to him, violates my human dignity."

Our argument takes the following form: We start from the common and uncontroversial idea that persons have a right to life that entails the right not to be killed as well as the right that others do not contribute to one's

---

[10] See Larry Alexander, "The Ontology of Consent," *Analytic Philosophy* 5, no. 1 (2014): 102–113.

killing.[11] These rights are part of the bundle of rights that we have over our own body. The normative powers to waive these rights belong to them—this is, as we have argued, part of the dignity of persons. Now, if a person waives her right to life by asking for assistance in dying, she thereby exercises her normative powers that are constitutive of her human dignity. As we have explained, this changes the deontic status of the action: Although it was impermissible to take any measures that lead to a person's death, it is now permissible to help her. To deny a person the power to make this action permissible means to disrespect her human dignity.

However, and we take this point to be an important contribution to the debate about assisted suicide, a person's request to be assisted in terminating her own life does not alone provide other persons with reasons or a duty to help her. As we have explained, the specific reasons why a person wants to waive a right are not essential to the exercise of her normative powers—she only needs to want to make the action permissible. By waiving rights, we do not create reasons speaking in favor of doing what is thereby made permissible. The waiving of a right thus cannot by itself provide other persons with reasons. Say, for instance, that the person had no reason to end her life. By waiving her right, she would not create a reason for another person to assist her in ending her life. Whether other persons *should* assist her in dying thus depends, in our view, on reasons that are not provided by appeals to human dignity (see below). In other words, although the exercise of normative powers can change the deontic status of actions, it does not create reasons for other persons to perform the action that is made permissible.

Locating the Argument within the Debate about Assisted Suicide

What are the advantages of this understanding of dignity in its practical role? First, because it is an account of human dignity that is plausible independently from any normative beliefs about the practice of assisted suicide, our argument avoids the instrumentalization of human dignity for specific (ideological) purposes. We regard this to be an important point in itself, but also because, especially with regard to controversial topics such as assisted suicide, it is quite common that human dignity is used in

---

[11] For an extensive discussion of the right to life and its relation to assisted death, see Joel Feinberg, "Voluntary Euthanasia and the Inalienable Right to Life," *Philosophy & Public Affairs* 7, no. 2 (1978): 93–123.

a rather vague way and is given no clear content. It is then employed as a conversation stopper and rhetorical device only. By contrast, in our argument, human dignity is given a specific content and assigned a distinct role in the debate about assisted suicide. This enables us to clarify the relation of human dignity to other arguments in the debate about assisted suicide.

On the one hand, we can distinguish our argument from what is commonly referred to as the "argument from autonomy." As we have shown, human dignity is different from autonomy in that the exercise of normative powers changes the deontic status of actions, whereas the autonomous will alone does not have this normative power. On this understanding, arguments to the effect that dignity means nothing else than respect for autonomy, and is thus redundant, can be rejected.[12] Furthermore, the relation of human dignity and autonomy is clarified: The exercise of one's normative powers has, of course, to be an autonomous choice. However, the moral permissibility of assisted suicide does not derive from the fact that a person's decision is autonomous. It is rather a person's exercise of her normative powers—that are tied to the rights that she has over her own body—that does the normative work. Our argument thus shows how autonomy and human dignity are different from each other and operate on different levels.[13]

On the other hand, the account we have developed allows us to identify the place and importance of other arguments, such as the "argument from mercy." Unbearable suffering and other conditions in which persons find themselves, and that often give rise to their request for assisted suicide, could be viewed as providing us with *reasons* (and possibly sometimes even with a duty) to help them terminate their own lives. They do not, however, make the acts in question permissible. This is what is done by the exercise of the normative power to release others from their duty not to assist someone in ending his or her life. This is the role that dignity can play in these situations; and it is the only role it can play. Dignity does not create reasons to assist others in ending their lives, it only makes them permissible; it does so when the relevant normative powers are exercised.

---

[12] See Macklin, "Dignity Is a Useless Concept," 1419f.

[13] For a different, and in our view less convincing, way to relate human dignity and autonomy, see Margaret Pabst Battin, "Suicide: A *Fundamental* Human Right?", in *The Least Worst Death* (New York: Oxford University Press, 1994), 277–288. Battin argues that the right to autonomy is a fundamental right that is rooted in human dignity, by which she wants to give the right to autonomy a special normative force.

One further merit that relates to our status-based account of dignity is the following: In contrast to accounts that regard human dignity as some kind of absolute value, our argument is not faced with the following common objection: It is sometimes held that if we qualify certain conditions of persons—such as unbearable suffering or the loss of control—as undignified, and if we appeal to such conditions as reasons for helping them to terminate their own lives, we thereby also devalue the lives of those persons who do not want to terminate their own lives.[14] But this admittedly problematic implication does not follow from our argument. After all, having human dignity is regarded as a status, and the act of making it permissible for others to help does not imply any statements about the value of lives at all.

It might be objected that our argument yields the conclusion that certain practices that are widely regarded as paradigmatic violations of human dignity, such as enslaving and torturing people, also have to be regarded as morally permissible if they are consented to. Because we also believe that persons have the normative power to waive their right to life, one could think that we also hold the view that we have the power to waive the right not to be enslaved or the right not to be tortured. This, however, does not follow from our account of dignity. Consider the example of consent slavery. As a slave, one would have no rights and no normative powers. We could only become slaves if we had the normative powers to get rid of our rights and powers. This is, however, impossible on our account. We can waive rights by exercising normative powers, but we cannot give up our rights by exercising our normative powers. We could, of course, consent to being completely dominated by another person, the possible slaveholder. But this waiving of rights could be withdrawn anytime we wanted to do so. This is incompatible with being someone who has no rights and powers anymore. Having dignity means being someone who has normative powers that cannot be waived. Thus, whatever amounts to a violation of dignity cannot be based on the exercise of normative powers. Rights can be waived, not the normative powers we have as beings with dignity.

<hr>

[14] See, for example, Chapter 3 in this volume.

BIBLIOGRAPHY

Alexander, Larry. "The Ontology of Consent." *Analytic Philosophy* 5, no. 1 (2014): 102–113.

"Americans Rank Alzheimer's as Most Feared Disease," November 13, 2012. Available at http://www.helpforalzheimersfamilies.com/alzheimers-dementia-care-services/alzheimers_feared_disease.

Anderson, Elizabeth. *Value in Ethics and Economics*. Cambridge, Mass.: Harvard University Press, 1993.

Anscombe, G. E. M. "The Dignity of the Human Being." In *Human Life, Action and Ethics. Essays by G.E.M. Anscombe*, edited by Mary Geach and Luke Gormally, 67–73. Charlottesville, Va.: Imprint Academic, 2005.

Aviv, Rachel. "The Death Treatment." *The New Yorker*, June 22, 2015. Available at http://www.newyorker.com/magazine/2015/06/22/the-death-treatment.

Battin, Margaret Pabst. "Assisted Suicide: What Can We Learn from Germany?" In *The Least Worst Death*, 254–270. New York: Oxford University Press, 1994.

Battin, Margaret Pabst. "Suicide: A *Fundamental* Human Right?" In *The Least Worst Death*, 277–288. New York: Oxford University Press, 1994.

Battin, Margaret Pabst. *The Least Worst Death: Essays in Bioethics on the End of Life*. New York: Oxford University Press, 1994.

Battin, Margaret Pabst. *Ending Life*. New York: Oxford University Press, 2005.

Battin, Margaret Pabst. "The Irony of Supporting Physician-Assisted Suicide: A Personal Account." *Medical Health Care and Philosophy* 13, no. 4 (2010): 403–411.

Battin, Margaret Pabst, ed. *The Ethics of Suicide: Historical Sources*. New York: Oxford University Press, 2015. Available at http://ethicsofsuicide.lib.utah.edu.

Beitz, Charles R. "Human Dignity in the Theory of Human Rights: Nothing But a Phrase?" *Philosophy and Public Affairs* 41, no. 3 (2013): 259–290.

Beyleveld, Deryck, and Roger Brownsword. *Human Dignity in Bioethics and Biolaw*. New York: Oxford University Press, 2001.

Bilefsky, Dan, and Christopher Schuetze. "Dutch Law Would Allow Assisted Suicide for Healthy Older People." *New York Times*, October 13, 2016. Available at http://www.nytimes.com/2016/10/14/world/europe/dutch-law-would-allow-euthanasia-for-healthy-elderly-people.html?_r=0.

Bird, Colin. "Dignity as a Moral Concept." *Social Philosophy & Policy* 30, no. 1–2 (2013): 150–176.

Blackstone, William T. "Human Rights and Human Dignity." *Philosophical Forum* 9, no. 1–2 (1971): 3–37.

Bouvia v. The Superior Court of Los Angeles County, 179 Cal.App.3d 1127 (1986).

Boyle, Joseph M., Germain Grisez, and Olaf Tollefsen. *Free Choice: A Self-Referential Argument*. Notre Dame, IN: University of Notre Dame Press, 1976.

Breitbart, W. "Depression, Hopelessness, and Desire for Hastened Death in Terminally Ill Patients with Cancer." *JAMA* 284, no. 22 (2000): 2907–2911.

Buss, Sarah. "Personal Autonomy." *The Stanford Encyclopedia of Philosophy*. Winter Edition, 2016. Available at https://plato.stanford.edu/archives/win2016/entries/personal-autonomy.

Chappell, Timothy D. J. *Understanding Human Goods: A Theory of Ethics*. Edinburgh, UK: Edinburgh University Press, 1998.

Chochinov, Harvey Max. "Dignity-Conserving Care—A New Model for Palliative Care: Helping the Patient Feel Valued." *JAMA* 287, no. 17 (2002): 2253–2260.

Chochinov, Harvey Max, Thomas Hack, Thomas Hassard, Linda J. Kristjanson, Susan McClement, and Mike Harlos. "Dignity in the Terminally Ill: A Cross-Sectional, Cohort Study." *The Lancet* 360, no. 9350 (2002): 2026–2030.

Chochinov, Harvey Max, Douglas Tataryn, Jennifer J. Clinch, and Deborah Dudgeon. "Will to Live in the Terminally Ill." *The Lancet* 354, no. 9181 (1999): 816–819.

Cholbi, Michael. "A Kantian Defense of Prudential Suicide." *Journal of Moral Philosophy* 7, no. 4 (2010): 489–515.

Cholbi, Michael. "Kant on Euthanasia and the Duty to Die: Clearing the Air." *Journal of Medical Ethics* 41, no. 8 (2015): 607–610.

Cholbi, Michael. *Understanding Kant's Ethics*. Cambridge: Cambridge University Press, 2016.

Cipolletta, Sabrina, and Nadia Oprandi. "What Is a Good Death? Health Care Professionals' Narrations on End-of-Life Care." *Death Studies* 38, no. 1 (2014): 20–27.

Cochrane, Alasdair. "Undignified Bioethics." *Bioethics* 24, no. 5 (2010): 234–241.

Cohen, Carl. "The Case for the Use of Animals in Biomedical Research." *New England Journal of Medicine* 315, no. 14 (1986): 78–80.

Coleman, Diane. "New Mexico Lower Court Parrots the Language and Platitudes of Assisted Suicide Advocacy Groups." *Not Dead Yet News & Commentary*, January 14, 2014. Available at http://notdeadyet.org/2014/01/new-mexico-lower-court-parrots-the-language-and-platitudes-of-assisted-suicide-advocacy-groups.html.

Darwall, Stephen. "Because I Want It." *Social Philosophy and Policy* 18, no. 2 (2001):129–153.

Darwall, Stephen. *Welfare and Rational Care*. Princeton, N.J.: Princeton University Press, 2002.

Darwall, Stephen. "Moore, Normativity, and Intrinsic Value." *Ethics* 113, no. 3 (2003): 468–489.

Darwall, Stephen. "Respect and the Second-Person Standpoint." *Proceedings and Addresses of the American Philosophical Association* 78, no. 2 (2004): 43–59.

Darwall, Stephen. *The Second-Person Standpoint*. Cambridge, Mass.: Harvard University Press, 2006.

Darwall, Stephen. "The Value of Autonomy and Autonomy of the Will." *Ethics* 116, no. 2 (2006): 263–284.

de Beaufort, Inez. "The View from Before." *American Journal of Bioethics* 7, no. 4 (2007): 57–66.

de Beaufort, Inez D., and Suzanne van der Vathorst. "Dementia and Assisted Suicide and Euthanasia." *Journal of Neurology* 263, no. 7 (2016): 1463–1467.

de Boer, Marike, Rose-Marie Droes, Cees Jonker, Jan A. Eefsting, and Cees Hertogh. "Advance Directives for Euthanasia in Dementia: Do Law-Based Opportunities Lead to More Euthanasia?" *Health Policy* 98, no. 2–3 (2010): 256–262.

de Boer, Marike E., Cees M. P. M. Hertogh, Rose-Marie Droes, Cees Jonker, and Jan A. Eefsting. "Advance Directives in Dementia: Issues of Validity and Effectiveness." *International Psychogeriatrics* 22, no. 2 (2010): 201–208.

de Melo-Martin, Inmaculada. "An Undignified Bioethics: There Is No Method in This Madness." *Bioethics* 26, no. 4 (2012): 224–230.

Dean, Richard. *The Value of Humanity in Kant's Moral Theory*. Oxford: Oxford University Press (2006).

Debes, Remy. "Dignity's Gauntlet." *Philosophical Perspectives* 23, no. 1 (2009): 45–78.

Des Pres, Terrence. *The Survivor: An Anatomy of Life in the Death Camps*. New York: Oxford University Press, 1976.

Devine, Philip E. *Natural Law Ethics*. Westport, Conn.: Greenwood Press, 2000.

Dilley, Stephen, and Nathan J. Palpant, eds. *Human Dignity in Bioethics: From Worldviews to the Public Square*. New York: Routledge, 2013.

Dresser, Rebecca. "Dworkin on Dementia: Elegant Theory, Questionable Policy." *Hastings Center Report* 27, no. 2 (1995): 34–42.

Dresser, Rebecca. "Dignity Can Be a Useful Concept in Bioethics." In *Bioethics, Public Moral Argument, and Social Responsibility*, edited by Nancy M. P. King and Michael J. Hyde, 45–54. New York: Routledge, 2012.

Dresser, Rebecca. "A Fate Worse Than Death? How Biomarkers for Alzheimer's Disease Could Affect End-of-Life Choices." *Indiana Health Law Review* 12, no. 2 (2015): 651–669.

Dresser, Rebecca. "Autonomy and Its Limits in End-of-Life Law." In *The Oxford Handbook of U.S. Healthcare Law*, edited by I. Glenn Cohen, Allison K. Hoffman, and William M. Sage, 399–417. New York: Oxford University Press, 2016.

Düwell, Marcus, Jens Braarvig, Roger Brownsword, and Dietmar Mieth, eds. *The Cambridge Handbook of Human Dignity: Interdisciplinary Perspectives*. Cambridge: Cambridge University Press, 2014.

Dworkin, Ronald. *Life's Dominion: An Argument about Abortion, Euthanasia, and Individual Freedom*. New York: Knopf, 1993.

Dworkin, Ronald, Thomas Nagel, Robert Nozick, John Rawls, and Judith Jarvis Thomson. "Assisted Suicide: The Philosophers' Brief." *New York Review of Books*, March 27, 1997: 41–47. Available at http://www.nybooks.com/articles/archives/1997/mar/27/assisted-suicide-the-philosophers-brief.

Eckholm, Erik. "New Mexico Judge Affirms Right to 'Aid in Dying'." *New York Times*, January 13, 2014: A16.

Epictetus. *Discourses of Epictetus*. Translated by George Long. New York: Appleton, 1904.

Fazel, Seema, Tony Hope, and Robin Jacoby. "Assessment of Competence to Complete Advance Directives: Validation of a Patient Centred Approach." *BMJ* 318 (1999): 493–97.

Feinberg, Joel. "The Nature and Value of Rights." *Journal of Value Inquiry* 4, no. 4 (1970): 243–257.

Feinberg, Joel. "Voluntary Euthanasia and the Inalienable Right to Life." *Philosophy & Public Affairs* 7, no. 2 (1978): 93–123.

Feser, Edward. "Kripke, Ross and the Immaterial Aspects of Thought." In *Neo-Scholastic Essays*, 217–253. South Bend, Ind.: St Augustine's Press, 2015.

Finnis, John. *Fundamentals of Ethics*. Oxford: Clarendon, 1983.

Finnis, John. "A Philosophical Case Against Euthanasia." In *Euthanasia Examined*, edited by John Keown, 23–35. Cambridge: Cambridge University Press, 1995.

Finnis, John. *Aquinas: Moral, Political and Legal Theory*. Oxford: Oxford University Press, 1998.

Finnis, John. "Euthanasia and Justice." In *Human Rights and Common Good. Collected Essays of John Finnis: Volume III*, 211–241. Oxford: Oxford University Press, 2011.

Finnis, John. *Human Rights and Common Good. Collected Essays of John Finnis: Volume III*. Oxford: Oxford University Press, 2011.

Finnis, John. *Natural Law and Natural Rights*, 2nd edition. Oxford: Oxford University Press, 2011.

Finnis, John, John M. Boyle, and Germain Grisez. *Nuclear Deterrence, Morality, and Realism*. Oxford: Clarendon, 1987.

FitzPatrick, William J. "The Practical Turn in Ethical Theory: Korsgaard's Constructivism, Realism, and the Nature of Normativity." *Ethics* 115, no. 4 (2005): 651–691.

FitzPatrick, William J. "Review of Richard Dean, *Value of Humanity in Kant's Moral Theory*." *Mind* 116, no. 464 (2007): 1098–1104.

Fletcher, Guy. "A Fresh Start for the Objective-List Theory of Well-Being." *Utilitas* 25, no. 2 (2013): 206–220.

Fukuyama, Francis. *Our Posthuman Future: Consequences of the Biotechnology Revolution*. New York: Farrar, Strauss and Giroux, 2002.

Ganzini, Linda, Elizabeth R. Goy, and Steven K. Dobscha, "Why Oregon Patients Request Assisted Death: Family Members' Views." *Journal of General Internal Medicine* 23, no. 2 (2008): 154–157.

Ganzini, Linda, Elizabeth R. Goy, and Steven K. Dobscha. "Oregonians' Reasons for Requesting Physician Aid in Dying." *Archives of Internal Medicine* 169, no. 5 (2009): 489–492.

Garrett, Mario. "Fear of Dementia." *iAge Blog*, May 11, 2013. Available at https://www.psychologytoday.com/blog/iage/201305/fear-dementia.

Gentzler, Jyl. "What Is a Death with Dignity?" *Journal of Medicine and Philosophy* 28, no. 4 (2003): 461–487.

Georges, Jean-Jacques, Bregje Onwuteaka-Philipsen, Martien T. Muller, Gerrit van der Wal, Agnes van der Heide, and Paul J. van der Maas. "Relatives' Perspective on the Terminally Ill Patients Who Died after Euthanasia or Physician-Assisted Suicide: A Retrospective Cross-Sectional Interview Study in the Netherlands." *Death Studies* 31, no. 1 (2007): 1–15.

Gewirth, Alan. *Self-Fulfillment*. Princeton, N.J.: Princeton University Press, 2009.

Gill, Carole J. "Health Professionals, Disability, and Assisted Suicide: An Examination of Relevant Empirical Evidence and Reply to Batavia." *Psychology, Public Policy and the Law*, 6 (2000): 526–545.

Gómez-Lobo, Alfons. *Morality and the Human Goods: An Introduction to Natural Law Ethics.* Washington, D.C.: Georgetown University Press, 2002.

Gormally, Luke, ed. *Euthanasia, Clinical Practice and the Law.* London: Linacre Centre, 1994.

Gormally, Luke. "Arguing from Autonomy and Dignity for the Legalization of Assistance in Suicide and Voluntary Euthanasia." *Acta Philosophica: Rivista Internazionale di Filosofia* 15, no. 2 (2006): 231–246.

Gormally, Luke. "The Good of Health and the Ends of Medicine." In *Natural Moral Law in Contemporary Society*, edited by Holger Zaborowski, 264–284. Washington, D.C.: Catholic University of America Press, 2010.

Gormally, Luke, David Albert Jones, and Roger Teichmann, eds. *The Moral Philosophy of Elizabeth Anscombe.* Exeter, UK: Imprint Academic, 2016.

Gorsuch, Neil. *The Future of Assisted Suicide and Euthanasia.* Princeton, N.J.: Princeton University Press, 2006.

Griffiths, John, Heleen Weyers, and Maurice Adams. *Euthanasia and Law in Europe.* Portland, Ore.: Hart Publishing, 2008.

Gunderson, Martin, and David Mayo. "Restricting Physician-Assisted Death to the Terminally Ill." *Hastings Center Report* 30, no. 6 (2000): 17–23.

Haddock, Jane. "Towards Further Clarification of the Concept 'Dignity'." *Journal of Advanced Nursing* 24, no. 5 (1996): 924–931.

Hasselmark, Berit. "The Selfish Suicide?" *World Right-to-Die Newsletter*, no. 65 (December 2013): 8. Available at http://www.worldrtd.net/sites/default/files/news-files/WRTD%20Newsletter%201213Web.pdf.

Häyry, Matti. "Another Look at Dignity." *Cambridge Quarterly of Healthcare Ethics* 13, no. 1 (2004): 7–14.

Heathwood, Chris. "Desire-Fulfillment Theory." In *The Routledge Handbook of Philosophy of Well-Being*, edited by Guy Fletcher, 135–147. London: Routledge, 2016.

Heggestad, Anne Kari T., Per Nortvedt, and Ashild Slettebo. "'Like a Prison without Bars': Dementia and Experiences of Dignity." *Nursing Ethics* 20, no. 8 (2013): 881–92.

Henig, Robin Marantz. "A Life or Death Situation." *The New York Times Magazine*, July 21, 2013. Available at http://www.nytimes.com/2013/07/21/magazine/a-life-or-death-situation.html.

Herman, Barbara. *The Practice of Moral Judgment.* Cambridge, Mass.: Harvard University Press, 1993.

Hertogh, Cees M. P. M. "The Role of Advance Euthanasia Directives as an Aid to Communication and Shared Decision-Making in Dementia." *Journal of Medical Ethics* 35, no. 2 (2009): 100–103.

Hertogh, Cees M. P. M., Marike E. de Boer, Rose-Marie Droes, and Jan A. Eefsting. "Would We Rather Lose Our Life Than Our Self? Lessons from the Dutch Debate on Euthanasia for Dementia Patients." *American Journal of Bioethics* 7, no. 4 (2007): 48–56.

Hertogh, Cees M. P. M., Marike E. de Boer, Rose-Marie Droes, and Jan A. Eefsting. "Beyond a Dworkinean View on Autonomy and Advance Directives in Dementia." *American Journal of Bioethics* 7, no. 4 (2007): W4–W6.

Heyer, Katharina. "Rejecting Rights: The Disability Critique of Physician Assisted Suicide." In *Special Issue Social Movements/Legal Possibilities*, edited by Austin Sarat, 77–112. Somerville, Mass.: Emerald Group, 2011.

Hill, Thomas. "Self-Regarding Suicide: A Modified Kantian View." *Suicide and Life–Threatening Behavior* 13, no. 4 (1983): 254–275.

Hill, Thomas. "Humanity as an End in Itself." In *Dignity and Practical Reason in Kant's Moral Theory*, 38–57. Ithaca, N.Y.: Cornell University Press, 1992.

Hill, Thomas. *Respect, Pluralism, and Justice*. Oxford: Oxford University Press, 2000.

Hills, Alison. "Rational Nature as the Source of Value." *Kantian Review* 10 (2005): 60–81.

Hohfeld, Wesley N. *Fundamental Legal Conceptions as Applied in Judicial Reasoning*, edited by D. Campbell and P. Thomas, with an introduction by N. E. Simmonds. Aldershot, UK: Ashgate, 2001.

Holy Bible, New International Version. Grand Rapids, Mich.: Zondervan, 1984.

Home Instead. "Americans Rank Alzheimer's as Most Feared Disease." November 13, 2012. Available at http://www.helpforalzheimersfamilies.com/alzheimers-dementia-care-services/alzheimers_feared_disease.

Hopkins, Brooke, and Peggy Battin. *Love under Trial*. Manuscript based on account at www.brookeandpeggy.blogspot.com.

Horton, Richard. "Rediscovering Human Dignity." *The Lancet* 364, no. 9439 (2004): 1081–1085.

Jacobson, Nora. "Dignity and Health: A Review." *Social Science and Medicine* 64, no. 2 (2006): 292–302.

Jacobson, Nora. "A Taxonomy of Dignity: A Grounded Theory Study." *BMC International Health and Human Rights* 9, no. 3 (2009). Available at https://doi.org/10.1186/1472-698X-9-3.

Jansen-van der Weide, Marijke C., Bregje D. Onwuteaka-Philipsen, and Gerrit van der Wal. "Granted, Undecided, Withdrawn, and Refused Requests for Euthanasia and Physician-Assisted Suicide." *Archives of Internal Medicine* 165, no. 15 (2005): 1698–1704.

Joerden, Jan C., Eric Hilgendorf, and Felix Thiele, eds. *Menschenwürde und Medizin: Ein interdisziplinäres Handbuch*. Berlin: Duncker & Humblot, 2013.

Joiner, Thomas. *Why People Die by Suicide*. Cambridge, Mass.: Harvard University Press, 2007.

Jordan, Matthew C. "Bioethics and 'Human Dignity'." *Journal of Medicine and Philosophy* 35, no. 2 (2010): 180–196.

Kaczor, Christopher. *A Defense of Dignity: Creating Life, Destroying Life, and Protecting the Rights of Conscience*. Notre Dame, Ind.: University of Notre Dame Press, 2013.

Kant, Immanuel. *Groundwork of the Metaphysics of Morals*. Translated by H. J. Paton. New York: Harper & Row, 1964.

Kant, Immanuel. *The Critique of Practical Reason*. Translated by Lewis White Beck. New York: Macmillan, 1985.

Kant, Immanuel. *The Metaphysics of Morals*. Translated by Mary Gregor. Cambridge: Cambridge University Press, 1991.

Kant, Immanuel. *Grounding for the Metaphysics of Morals. With on a Supposed Right to Lie Because of Philanthropic Concerns*. Translated by James W. Ellington, 3rd edition. Indianapolis, Ind.: Hackett, 1993.

Kant, Immanuel. *Practical Philosophy*. Edited and translated by Mary J. Gregor. Cambridge: Cambridge University Press, 1996.

Kant, Immanuel. *Groundwork of the Metaphysics of Morals*. Edited by Mary Gregor and Jens Timmerman. Cambridge: Cambridge University Press, 1998.

Kant, Immanuel. *Lectures on Ethics*. Edited by J. B. Schneewind, translated by Peter Heath. Cambridge: Cambridge University Press, 2001.

Kant, Immanuel. *Groundwork of the Metaphysics of Morals*. Edited by Mary Gregor and Jens Timmermann, revised edition. Cambridge: Cambridge University Press, 2012.

Karlawish, J. H. T., D. J. Cassarett, B. D. James, S. X. Xie, and S. Y. H. Kim. "The Ability of Persons with Alzheimer Disease (AD) to Make a Decision about Taking an AD Treatment." *Neurology* 64, no. 9 (2005): 1514–1519.

Kateb, George. *Human Dignity*. Cambridge, Mass.: Harvard University Press, 2011.

Kaufmann, Paulus, Hannes Kuch, Christiane Neuhaeuser, and Elaine Webster, eds. *Humiliation, Degradation, Dehumanization: Human Dignity Violated*. Dordrecht: Springer, 2010.

Keown, John. "Restoring the Sanctity of Life and Replacing the Caricature: A Reply to David Price." *Legal Studies* 26, no. 1 (2006): 109–119.

Keown, John. *The Law and Ethics of Medicine: Essays on the Inviolability of Human Life*. New York: Oxford University Press, 2012.

Keown, John. "A New Father for Law and Ethics of Medicine." In *Reason, Morality, and Law: The Philosophy of John Finnis*, edited by John Keown and Robert P. George, 290–307. Oxford: Oxford University Press, 2013.

Killmister, Suzy. "Dignity: Not Such a Useless Concept." *Journal of Medical Ethics* 36, no. 3 (2009): 160–164.

Killmister, Suzy. "Dignity: Personal, Social, Human." *Philosophical Studies* (2016). Available at http://link.springer.com/article/10.1007/s11098-016-0788-y.

Kim, Scott Y. H., Raymond de Vries, and John R. Peteet. "Euthanasia and Assisted Suicide of Patients with Psychiatric Disorders in the Netherlands 2011 to 2014." *JAMA Internal Medicine* 73, no. 4 (2016): 362–368.

Kirchhoffer, David G. *Human Dignity in Contemporary Bioethics*. Amherst, N.Y.: Teneo Press, 2013.

Kitwood, Tom, and Kathleen Bredin. "Towards a Theory of Dementia Care: Personhood and Well-Being." *Ageing & Society* 12, no. 3 (1992): 269–287.

Klein, David Alan. "Medical Disparagement of the Disability Experience: Empirical Evidence for the 'Expressivist Objection'." *AJOB Primary Research* 2, no. 2 (2011): 8–20.

Kleinfield, N. R. "Fraying at the Edges." Special Section, *New York Times*, May 1, 2016.

Klonsky, E. David, Roman Kotov, Shelly Bakst, Jonathan Rabinowitz, and Evelyn J. Bromet. "Hopelessness as a Predictor of Attempted Suicide among First Admission Patients with Psychosis: A 10-Year Cohort Study." *Suicide and Life-Threatening Behavior* 41, no. 1 (2012): 1–10.

Korsgaard, Christine. *Creating the Kingdom of Ends*. Cambridge: Cambridge University Press, 1996.

Korsgaard, Christine. "Kant's Formula of Humanity." In *Creating the Kingdom of Ends*, 106–132. Cambridge: Cambridge University Press, 1996.

Korsgaard, Christine. *The Sources of Normativity*. Cambridge: Cambridge University Press, 1996.

Lee, Patrick, and Robert P. George. *Body–Self Dualism in Contemporary Ethics and Politics*. New York: Cambridge University Press, 2007.

Lee, Patrick, and Robert P. George. "The Nature and Basis of Human Dignity." *Ratio Juris* 21, no. 2 (2008): 173–193.

Lindsay, Ronald A. "Oregon's Experience: Evaluating the Record." *American Journal of Bioethics* 9, no. 3 (2009): 19–27.

Luban, David. "Human Dignity, Humiliation, and Torture." *Kennedy Institute of Ethics Journal* 19, no. 3 (2009): 211–230.

MacCormick, Neil, and Joseph Raz. "Voluntary Obligations and Normative Powers." *Proceedings of the Aristotelian Society: Supplementary Volumes* 46, no. 1 (1972): 59–102.

Macklin, Ruth. "Dignity Is a Useless Concept." *BMJ* 327, no. 7429 (2003): 1419–1420.

Macklin, Ruth. "Reflections on the Human Dignity Symposium: Is Dignity a Useless Concept?" *Journal of Palliative Care* 20, no. 3 (2004): 212–216.

Malpas, Jeff, and Norelle Lickiss, eds. *Perspectives on Human Dignity.* Dordrecht: Springer, 2007.

Mappes, Thomas. "Some Reflections on Advance Directives." *APA Newsletters: Newsletter on Philosophy and Medicine* 98, no. 1 (1998): 106–111.

Mattson, David J., and Susan G. Clark. "Human Dignity in Concept and Practice." *Policy Sciences* 44, no. 4 (2011): 303–319.

McCrudden, Christopher. "Human Dignity and Judicial Interpretation of Human Rights." *European Journal of International Law* 19, no. 4 (2008): 655–724.

McCrudden Christopher, ed. *Understanding Human Dignity.* Oxford: Oxford University Press, 2014.

McMahan, Jeff. *The Ethics of Killing: Problems at the Margins of Life.* New York: Oxford University Press, 2002.

McMahan, Jeff. "An Alternative to Brain Death." *Journal of Law, Medicine and Ethics* 34, no. 1 (2006): 44–48.

McMahan, Jeff. "Killing Embryos for Stem Cell Research." *Metaphilosophy* 38, no. 2–3 (2007): 170–189.

McPherson, Christine J., Keith G. Wilson, and Mary Ann Murray. "Feeling Like a Burden: Exploring the Perspectives of Patients at the End of Life." *Social Science & Medicine* 64, no. 2 (2007): 417–427.

Mead, Rebecca. "The Sense of an Ending." *The New Yorker*, May 20, 2013: 92–103.

Meilaender, Gilbert. *Neither Beast Nor God: The Dignity of the Human Person.* New York: Encounter Books, 2009.

Menzell, Paul, and Bonnie Steinbock. "Advance Directives, Dementia, and Physician-Assisted Death." *Journal of Law, Medicine & Ethics* 41, no. 2 (2013): 484–500.

Metz, Thaddeus. "African Conceptions of Human Dignity: Vitality and Community as the Ground of Human Rights." *Human Rights Review* 13, no. 1 (2012): 19–37.

Meyers, Michael. "Dignity, Rights, and Self-Control." *Ethics* 99, no. 3 (1989): 520–534.

Morita, Tatsuya, Yukihiro Sakaguchi, Kei Hirai, Satoru Tsuneto, and Yasuo Shima. "Desire for Death and Requests to Hasten Death of Japanese Terminally Ill Cancer Patients Receiving Specialized Inpatient Palliative Care." *Journal of Pain and Symptom Management* 27, no. 1 (2004): 44–52.

Muders, Sebastian. "Natural Good Theories and the Value of Human Dignity." *Cambridge Quarterly of Healthcare Ethics* 25, no. 2 (2016), 239–249.

Muders, Sebastian. "Human Dignity in Bioethics." *Encyclopedia of Life Sciences* (2017). Available at http://www.els.net/WileyCDA/ElsArticle/refId-a0027020.html.

Müller, Anselm W. "Radical Subjectivity: Morality versus Utilitarianism." *Ratio* 19, no. 2 (1977): 115–132.

Murphy, Mark C. *Natural Law and Practical Rationality.* New York: Cambridge University Press, 2001.

Neuhäuser, Christian, and Ralf Stoecker. "Human Dignity as Universal Nobility." In *The Cambridge Handbook of Human Dignity: Interdisciplinary Perspectives*, edited by Marcus Düwell, Jens Braarvig, Roger Brownsword, and Dietmar Mieth, 298–309. Cambridge: Cambridge University Press, 2014.

Nhat Hanh, Thich. *Vietnam: Lotus in a Sea of Fire.* Foreword by Thomas Merton. New York: Hill and Wang, 1967.

Nordenfelt, Lennart. "The Varieties of Dignity." *Health Care Analysis* 12, no. 2 (2004): 83–89.

Nuffield Council on Bioethics. "Dementia: Ethical Issues" (2009). Available at http://nuffieldbioethics.org/dementia.

Nussbaum, Martha Craven. *Women and Human Development: The Capabilities Approach.* New York: Cambridge University Press, 2001.

Nussbaum, Martha Craven. *Frontiers of Justice: Disability, Nationality, Species Membership.* Cambridge, Mass.: Belknap, 2007.

Nussbaum, Martha Craven. "The Capabilities of People with Cognitive Disabilities." *Metaphilosophy* 40, no. 3–4 (2009): 331–351.

Parfit, Derek. *On What Matters, Volume One.* Oxford: Oxford University Press, 2011.

Parfit, Derek. *On What Matters, Volume Two.* Oxford: Oxford University Press, 2011.

Paterson, Graig. *Physician-Assisted Suicide and Euthanasia: A Natural Law Ethics Approach.* Aldershot, UK: Ashgate, 2008.

Pinker, Steven. "The Stupidity of Dignity." *The New Republic* 238, May 28, 2008: 28–31. Available at https://newrepublic.com/article/64674/the-stupidity-dignity.

Planned Parenthood of Southeastern Pa. v. Casey, 505 U.S. 833 (1992).

Post, Stephen. "Physician-Assisted Suicide in Alzheimer's Disease." *Journal of the American Geriatrics Society* 45, no. 5 (1997): 647–651.

Pullman, Daryl. "Death, Dignity, and Moral Nonsense." *Journal of Palliative Care* 20, no. 3 (2004): 171–178.

Quinn, Warren. "Actions, Intentions, and Consequences: The Doctrine of Double Effect." *Philosophy and Public Affairs* 18, no. 4 (1989): 334–351.

Rabins, Peter. "Can Suicide Be a Rational and Ethical Act in Persons with Early or Pre-dementia?" *American Journal of Bioethics* 7, no. 6 (2007): 47–49.

Rachels, James. *Created from Animals: The Moral Implications of Darwinism.* Oxford: Oxford University Press, 1990.

Regan, Tom. *The Case for Animal Rights.* London: Routledge and Keegan Paul, 1983.

Report of the House of Lords Select Committee on Medical Ethics, HL Paper 21-1 of 1993-94. London: HMSO, 1994.

Rosen, Michael. *Dignity: Its History and Meaning.* Cambridge, Mass.: Harvard University Press, 2012.

Ross, James. *Thought and World. The Hidden Necessities.* Notre Dame, Ind.: University of Notre Dame Press, 2008.

Sabat, Steven. "Voices of Alzheimer's Disease Sufferers: A Call for Treatment Based on Personhood." *Journal of Clinical Ethics* 9, no. 1 (1998): 35–48.

Sabat, Steven. "The Person with Dementia as Understood through Stern's Critical Personalism." In *Beyond Loss: Dementia, Identity, Personhood*, edited by Lars-Christer

Hyden, Hilde Lindemann, and Jens Brockmeier, 24–38. New York: Oxford University Press, 2014.

Saigal, Saroj, Barbara L. Stoskopf, David Feeny, William Furlong, Elizabeth Burrows, Peter L. Rosenbaum, and Lorraine Hoult. "Differences in Preferences for Neonatal Outcomes among Health Care Professionals, Parents, and Adolescents." *JAMA* 281, no. 21 (1999): 1991–1997.

Scanlon, Thomas M. *What We Owe to Each Other*. Cambridge, Mass.: Belknap, 1998.

Schaber, Peter. *Instrumentalisierung und Würde*. Paderborn, Germany: Mentis, 2010.

Schaber, Peter. "Menschenwürde: Ein für die Medizinethik irrelevanter Begriff?" *Ethik in der Medizin* 24, no. 4 (2012): 297–306.

Schaber, Peter. "Würde als Status." In *Menschenwürde. Eine philosophische Debatte über Dimensionen ihrer Kontingenz*. Edited by Eva Weber-Guskar and Mario Brandhorst. Berlin: Suhrkamp, 2017.

Schiller, Friedrich. *On Grace and Dignity*. Translated by George Gregory. Washington, D.C.: Schiller Institute, [1793] 1992.

Schroeder, Doris. "Dignity: Two Riddles and Four Concepts." *Cambridge Quarterly of Healthcare Ethics* 17, no. 1 (2008): 230–238.

Schroeder, Doris. "Dignity: One, Two, Three, Four, Five, Still Counting." *Cambridge Quarterly of Healthcare Ethics* 19, no. 1 (2010): 118–125.

Schüklenk, Udo, Johannes J. M. van Delden, Jocelyn Downie, Sheila A. M. Mclean, Ross Upshur, and Daniel Weinstock. "End-of-Life Decision-Making in Canada: The Report by the Royal Society of Canada Expert Panel on End-of-Life Decision-Making." *Bioethics* 25, no. s1 (2011): 1–73.

Seligman, Martin. *Helplessness: On Depression, Development, and Death*. New York: Freeman, 1992.

Sensen, Oliver. *Kant on Human Dignity*. Berlin: De Gruyter, 2011.

Sheldon, Tony. "Dementia Patient's Suicide Was Lawful, Say Dutch Authorities." *BMJ* 343 (2011): 7510.

Simpson, Evan. "Harms to Dignity, Bioethics, and the Scope of Biolaw." *Journal of Palliative Care* 20, no. 3 (2004): 185–200.

Singer, Peter. *Practical Ethics*, 2nd edition. Cambridge: Cambridge University Press, 1993.

Smart, J. J. C., and J. J. Haldane. *Atheism and Theism*. Oxford: Blackwell, 1996.

Smith, Stephen W. *End-of-Life Decisions in Medical Care: Principles and Policies for Regulating the Dying Process*. Cambridge: Cambridge University Press, 2012.

Snijdewind, Marianne, C. Dick L. Willems, Luc Deliens, Bregje D. Onwuteaka-Phillipsen, and Kenneth Chambaere. "A Study of the First Year of the End-of-Life Clinic for Physician-Assisted Dying in the Netherlands." *JAMA Internal Medicine* 175, no. 10 (2015): 1633–1640.

Spaemann, Robert. *Love and the Dignity of Human Life*. Grand Rapids, Mich.: Eerdmans, 2012.

Spiegelberg, Herbert. "Human Dignity: A Challenge to Contemporary Philosophy." *Philosophical Forum* 9, no. 1–2 (1971): 39–64.

Steinhauser, Karen E., Elizabeth C. Clipp, Maya McNeilly, Nicholas A. Christakis, Lauren M. McIntyre, and James A. Tulsky. "In Search of a Good Death: Observations of Patients, Families, and Providers." *Annals of Internal Medicine* 132, no. 10 (2000): 825–832.

Stoecker, Ralf. "Three Crucial Turns on the Road to an Adequate Understanding of Human Dignity." In *Violations of Human Dignity*, edited by Paulus Kaufmann, Hannes Kuch, Christian Neuhäuse, and Elaine Webster, 7–19. Dordrecht: Springer, 2010.

Strawson, Peter Frederick. *Freedom and Resentment and Other Essays*. London: Routledge, 2008.

Sulmasy, Daniel. "Dignity and Bioethics: History, Theory, and Selected Applications." In *Human Dignity and Bioethics*, edited by Adam Schulman, Edmund D. Pellegrino, and Thomas W. Merrill, 469–501. Washington, D.C.: US Independent Agencies and Commissions, 2008.

Sumner, Leonard W. *Welfare, Happiness, and Ethics*. Oxford: Clarendon, 1996.

Sumner, Leonard W. *Assisted Death: A Study in Ethics and Law*. New York: Oxford University Press, 2011.

Sussman, David. "What's Wrong with Torture?" *Philosophy & Public Affairs* 33, no. 1 (2005): 1–33.

Tasioulas, John. "Human Dignity and the Foundations of Human Rights." In *Understanding Human Dignity*, edited by Christopher McCrudden, 291–312. Oxford: Oxford University Press, 2013.

United Nations. *Universal Declaration of Human Rights*. New York: United Nations, 1948. Available at http://www.un.org/en/universal-declaration-human-rights.

Vacco v. Quill, 521 U.S. 793 (1997).

Valerius Maximus. *Memorable Doings and Sayings*, Book II. Edited and translated by D. R. Shackleton Bailey. Cambridge, Mass.: Harvard University Press, 2000.

van Alphen, Jojanneke E., Ge A. Donker, and Richard L. Marquet. "Requests for Euthanasia in General Practice before and after Implementation of the Dutch Euthanasia Act." *British Journal of General Practice* 60, no. 573 (2010): 263–267.

van der Graaf, Rieke, and Johannes J. M. van Delden. "Clarifying Appeals to Dignity in Medical Ethics from an Historical Perspective." *Bioethics* 23, no. 3 (2009): 151–160.

Velleman, J. David. "A Right of Self-Termination?" *Ethics* 109, no. 3 (1999): 606–628.

Velleman, J. David. "Love as a Moral Emotion." *Ethics* 109, no. 2 (1999): 338–374.

Waldron, Jeremy. *Dignity, Rank, and Rights*. New York: Oxford University Press, 2012.

Waldron, Jeremy. *The Harm in Hate Speech*. Cambridge, Mass.: Harvard University Press, 2012.

Waldron, Jeremy. "Is Dignity the Foundation of Human Rights?" In *Philosophical Foundations of Human Rights*, edited by Rowan Cruft, Matthew Liao, and Massimo Renzo, 117–137. Oxford: Oxford University Press, 2015.

Walker-Robinson, Sarah. *Let's Talk (Some More) about Dementia*. June 17, 2014. Available at http://nuffieldbioethics.org/blog/lets-talk-some-more-about-dementia.

Williams, Bernard. "The Makropulos Case: Reflections on the Tedium of Immortality." In *Problems of the Self*, 82–100. Cambridge: Cambridge University Press, 1973.

Wood, Allen W. "Kant on Duties Regarding Nonrational Nature." *Proceedings of the Aristotelian Society Supplementary Volume* 72, no. 1 (1998): 189–210.

Wood, Allen W. *Kant's Ethical Thought*. Cambridge: Cambridge University Press (1999).

Wood, Allen W. *Kantian Ethics*. Cambridge: Cambridge University Press, 2007.

Woods, B. "The Legacy of Professor Tom Kitwood 1937–1998." *Aging & Mental Health* 3, no. 1 (1999): 5–7.

INDEX OF PERSONS

INDEX OF SUBJECTS